Cambridge History of Medicine

EDITORS: CHARLES WEBSTER AND CHARLES ROSENBERG

Victorian lunacy

OTHER BOOKS IN THIS SERIES

Charles Webster, ed.   *Health, medicine, and mortality in the sixteenth century*
Ian Maclean   *The Renaissance notion of woman*
Michael MacDonald   *Mystical Bedlam*
Robert E. Kohler   *From medical chemistry to biochemistry*
Walter Pagel   *Joan Baptista Van Helmont*
Nancy Tomes   *A generous confidence*
Roger Cooter   *The cultural meaning of popular science*
Anne Digby   *Madness, morality, and medicine*
Roy Porter, ed.   *Patients and practitioners*
Guenter B. Risse   *Hospital life in Enlightenment Scotland*
Ann G. Carmichael   *Plague and the poor in early Renaissance Florence*

Victorian lunacy

*Richard M. Bucke and the practice
of late nineteenth-century psychiatry*

S.E.D. Shortt
*Department of History and Department of Family Medicine
Queen's University, Canada*

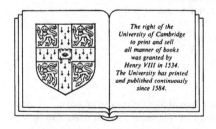

The right of the
University of Cambridge
to print and sell
all manner of books
was granted by
Henry VIII in 1534.
The University has printed
and published continuously
since 1584.

CAMBRIDGE UNIVERSITY PRESS

CAMBRIDGE
LONDON   NEW YORK   NEW ROCHELLE
MELBOURNE   SYDNEY

CAMBRIDGE UNIVERSITY PRESS
Cambridge, New York, Melbourne, Madrid, Cape Town, Singapore,
São Paulo, Delhi, Dubai, Tokyo, Mexico City

Cambridge University Press
The Edinburgh Building, Cambridge CB2 8RU, UK

Published in the United States of America by Cambridge University Press, New York

www.cambridge.org
Information on this title: www.cambridge.org/9780521172820

First published 1986
First paperback edition 2010

A catalogue record for this publication is available from the British Library

Library of Congress Cataloguing in Publication data
Shortt, S. E. D. (Samuel Edward Dole), 1947–
    Victorian lunacy.
    (Cambridge history of medicine)
    1. Psychiatric hospitals–Ontario–History–19th
century. 2. London Asylum for Insane (Ont.)–
History–19th century. 3. Bucke, Richard Maurice,
1837–1902. 4. Physicians–Ontario–Biography.
I. Title. II. Series. [DNLM: 1. Bucke, Richard
Maurice, 1837–1902. 2. Hospitals, Psychiatric–history
–Ontario. 3. London Asylum for Insane (Ont.)
4. Psychiatry–biography. 5. Psychiatry–History–
Ontario. WZ 100 B922S]
RC448.O53S56 1986 362.2'1'09713 85–26919

ISBN 978-0-521-30999-8 Hardback
ISBN 978-0-521-17282-0 Paperback

The wonderful phenomena of lunacy – what does that mean? Has it a physical basis? or physical entanglements? or what: It is a lesson to see Bucke's asylum at London – the hundreds on hundreds of his insane. I used to wander through the wards quite freely – go everywhere – even among the boisterous patients – the very violent. But I couldn't stand it long – I finally told Doctor I could not continue to do it. I think I gave him back the key which he had entrusted to me: It became a too-near fact – too poignant – too sharply painful – too ghastly true.

Walt Whitman
July, 1888

CONTENTS

List of tables	*page*	viii
List of illustrations		ix
Preface		xi
Abbreviations		xiv
Note on primary sources		xv
Introduction		I
1 The topography of a Victorian medical life		4
2 The human ecology of the London Asylum		26
3 Toward a secular physiology of mind		63
4 The social genesis of etiological speculation		94
5 Treatment tactics and professional aspirations		124
Epilogue		160
Notes		163
Index		205

TABLES

2.1   Asylum populations in Ontario and at London, selected years   39

2.2   Expenditures, London and Ontario Asylums, 1868–93   40

2.3   Asylum expenditures and total provincial expenditures, selected years   40

2.4   Turnover in London Asylum attendants, 1877–97   47

2.5   Assigned causes of insanity on admission, selected years   52

2.6   Duration of patient incarceration, selected years   52

2.7   Patient characteristics compared by percentage to Ontario population, selected years   53

2.8   Age of patients admitted to London Asylum, compared to distribution of ages in Ontario, by percentage, selected years   54

2.9   County of residence, London Asylum admissions, selected years   55

2.10   London Asylum expenditures and income from pay patients, selected years   56

2.11   Asylum admissions and discharges, selected years   60

5.1   Yearly reported results of gynecological surgery at the London Asylum, 1895–1900   144

5.2   Gynecological disorders diagnosed   148

5.3   Characteristics of gynecological and age-matched control patients, London Asylum, 1895–1900   149

5.4   Postsurgical course of gynecological patients   150

5.5   Discharge status of gynecological and control patients   150

5.6   Duration of stay for gynecological and control patients   151

5.7   Principal gynecological procedures   157

ILLUSTRATIONS

1 The Bucke family farm, c. 1840   5
2 Medical Faculty, McGill University, Côté Street, c. 1858   7
3 Montreal General Hospital, 1850s   8
4 Anatomy class, n.d., likely McGill University, c. 1860   10
5 Office occupied by R. M. Bucke's medical practice in Sarnia, Ontario, during the 1860s   17
6 R. M. Bucke, c. 1876   27
7 London Asylum, 1871   28
8 Medical Superintendent's house, London Asylum, n.d. (c. 1880)   29
9 Female ward, London Asylum, c. 1911   31
10 Title page and neurological illustrations from *Man's Moral Nature* (1879)   81
11 Title page from *Cosmic Consciousness* (1901)   110
12 R. M. Bucke in the library of his London Asylum office, 1899   114
13 Patients working on the London Asylum farm, n.d.   132
14 London Asylum Drama Group, c. 1885   134
15 London Asylum cricket team, 1895   135

PREFACE

Several years ago I had the pleasure of presenting a historio-graphical paper at an American university. I emphasized what I took to be something of a historical cliché: Written history is the subjective creation of the historian's mind rather than an objective replication of the past. Among those in the audience was an epidemiologist, himself an amateur historian, who refused to accept this view of history. Historians, he believed, were empiricists concerned only with establishing "what actually happened in the past." This struck me as a peculiar argument from an epidemiologist, a member of a discipline that devotes immense energy to scrutinizing clinical trials so as to expose or exclude the many commonly recognized sources of subjectivity and covert bias. Yet the pervasiveness of this viewpoint was reinforced several months later when I presented some of the material (which appears here as Chapter 4) to an audience of psychiatrists. During the discussion that followed, one of their number, reputed among his colleagues for an interest in history, accused me of being "biased." As he elaborated, it became clear that my misdemeanor was that I had departed from "the facts," that I had imposed upon my data my own analytical perspective. Twice damned for the same crime, I left this lecture unregenerate but aware that my viewpoint, at least among physicians, was far from the truism I had naively imagined.

In view of this possible source of controversy, it seems reasonable to make explicit three points. The first concerns the primary role of the historian. What distinguishes the historian from the antiquarian is not archival diligence, essential though this certainly is, but the construction he or she places upon the research material. With all the bias and preconception that this implies, history is, in short, nothing more than interpretation. The second point is less easily articulated, but has to do with my own beliefs about the way society works. Human communities are defined by a hierarchy of affluence and power in which those at the top have an interest in maintaining existing social relationships, while those at the bottom have an incentive for change. The arguments marshaled in the ongoing conflict between these polarities express divergent values which are determined, to a significant degree, by the economic and consequent social circumstances of their proponents. This view I consider as commonsensical rather than doctrinaire, but this time with the foreknowledge that what I perceive as a truism may well be rejected by others as incomprehensible. Finally, I would not wish those physicians to whom my views are unpalatable to dismiss this book with the accusation that I am simply "antipsychiatry"; on the contrary, I have the greatest respect for the humane psychiatric clinician. The object of this study is not to assign blame, but rather to foster critical insight.

It is a pleasure to acknowledge those individuals who have expedited my research and writing. Barbara L. Craig of the Ontario Archives shared with me her wide knowledge of government health records and ensured that they were available for expeditious perusal when required. Beth Miller of the Rare Book Room at the University of Western Ontario performed a similar function in placing at my disposal the materials of the Richard M. Bucke Collection. At the London Psychiatric Hospital, Mr. Charles Scott allowed me to examine records and photographs in the recently created replica of Bucke's study. Similar courtesies were extended by the Library of Congress and the McGill University Archives, as well as by a number of repositories in the United States and Great Britain to whom enquiries were addressed. The staff of the Bracken Library at Queen's University, and particularly of the Inter-Library Loan Department, have been a constant source of assistance during my research. Finally, I am particularly indebted to the Ontario Ministry of Health for permission to examine the records of the London Asylum, and to Mrs. Ida Moss for permission to quote from the correspondence of her grandfather, Richard M. Bucke.

Statistics for Chapter 5 were gathered by two diligent historians, Catherine A. Sims and James DeJonge. Computer assistance was patiently provided by Mr. Bill Ross of Queen's University Statlab. My colleagues in Family Medicine, Drs. John Anderson and Ron Lees, shared with me their knowledge of epidemiology and the analysis of clinical trials. While I alone am responsible for the final form in which Chapter 5 is cast, I appreciate the help of these various individuals.

I have been particularly fortunate in having two colleagues and friends who have taken an interest in the gestation of this volume. First, Thomas E. Brown has generously shared with me both his vast bibliographical knowledge of the history of psychiatry and his enthusiasm for long discussions on esoteric points of research. Without his stimulus over the last three years this book would have adopted a much different and, I am certain, less satisfactory form. Secondly, George Rawlyk has brought to bear on the evolving manuscript his astute editorial judgment. Despite his numerous other commitments he has always willingly read my material and offered his own important insights. In addition to these two scholars, I have discussed in conversation and correspondence aspects of this work with Paul Wood, Toby Gelfand, Bill Bynum, Andrew Scull, Roger Cooter, Colin Howell, Charles Rosenberg, and John Harrison, and from all of them, in important but often elusive ways, have learned more of my subject.

I appreciate financial support from the Advisory Research Committee of Queen's University and from the Social Science and Humanities Research Council of Canada. The manuscript was rapidly and accurately typed by Mrs. Marjorie Jeffrey who, in the process, stimulated my interest in the miracle of the word processor. Formatic order was brought to chaotic footnotes by the diligence of Mr. Allen Robertson.

Finally, my wife, Dr. Meri Bukowskyj, has patiently tolerated my excursion into the history of psychiatry and has rewarded me by sharing the nuance of her own research in clinical respirology. It has made for some profoundly esoteric dinner table non sequiturs of the type that only two research careers can share and enjoy.

ABBREVIATIONS

AJI	*American Journal of Insanity*
ARMS	Annual Report of the Medical Superintendent, London Asylum, Appendix to the Report of the Inspector for Prisons and Public Charities, Ontario Sessional Papers.
AS	London Asylum Scrapbooks, found in RMBC.
BHM	*Bulletin of the History of Medicine.*
FCB	Ontario Archives, Female Casebooks, London Asylum, R.G. 10, 2-C-1.
IC	Ontario Archives, Correspondence of the Inspector of Prisons and Public Charities, R.G. 10, 2-A-1.
IMB	Inspector's Minute Book, found in RMBC.
IR	Report of the Inspector for Prisons and Public Charities, Ontario Sessional Papers.
JHMAS	*Journal of the History of Medicine and Allied Sciences*
LC	Library of Congress, Manuscript Division, Washington, D.C.
LPH	London Psychiatric Hospital, formerly the London Asylum.
MCB	Ontario's Archives, Male Casebooks, London Asylum, R.G. 10, 2-C-1.
MH	*Medical History.*
MSJ	Medical Superintendent's Journal, found in RMBC.
MSOB	Medical Superintendent's Order Book, found in RMBC.
MUA	McGill University Archives.
RMBC	Richard Maurice Bucke Collection, D. B. Weldon Library, University of Western Ontario, London, Ontario, Canada

NOTE ON PRIMARY SOURCES

The major repository for materials relating directly to Richard
M. Bucke is the Rare Book Room at the D.B. Weldon Library,
University of Western Ontario, London, Canada. In addition to
voluminous correspondence with individuals such as H.B. Forman, Walt Whitman, Horace Traubel, and a scattering of other
individuals such as Edward Carpenter, this collection also contains Bucke's diaries covering the period from 1862 to 1868.
Bucke's medical casebooks and ledgers covering the period of his
general practice in Sarnia from 1865 to 1872 have been preserved
but, more significantly, the collection also contains the Journal of
the London Medical Superintendent for 1877 to 1884 and the
Medical Superintendent's Order Book for 1879 to 1890. In the
collection are drafts of Bucke's speeches, copies of many of his
publications, scrapbooks compiled by the asylum for the period
1877 to 1893 and the diary of Dr. Charles A. Sippi, the asylum
bursar from 1893 to 1897. An essential guide to this collection is
*Richard Maurice Bucke, A Catalogue Based on the Collections of the
University of Western Ontario Libraries,* edited by Mary Ann Jameson (London, Canada: University of Western Ontario, 1978).
This repository, then, provides a chronology of Bucke's career
and personal relationships, together with essential information on
his experience as a general practitioner and his activities as an
asylum superintendent.

The second major collection essential to this study is the Archives of the Province of Ontario. The correspondence of the
Inspector of Prisons and Public Charities (R.G. 10, 2-A-1) contains essential information on topics such as the regulations for
the daily administration of the asylums; activities of attendants
and assistant physician; patients, with particular references to
misdeeds and finances; newspaper publicity; and, finally, the ac-

tivities of the medical superintendent himself. The papers of the London Asylum (RG-10, 20-C-1 to 3-G) include male and female casebooks from 1870 to 1906, and a series of important registers dating from 1870 recording information such as the names of employees and attendants together with the dates of their tenure. An essential complement to this collection of material is found in the annual *Sessional Papers of the Province of Ontario* which contain the Report of the Inspector of Prisons and Public Charities and the yearly Report of the Medical Superintendent of the London Asylum during Bucke's entire asylum career.

Of published primary material, the most important sources are the various papers published by Bucke in the *American Journal of Insanity* between 1877 and 1900 and two of his books, *Man's Moral Nature* (New York: G.P. Putnam's Sons; Toronto: Willing & Williamson, 1879) and *Cosmic Consciousness: A Study in the Evolution of the Human Mind* (Philadelphia: Innes & Sons, 1901). To place this published material in context it is necessary to read widely in neuropsychiatric periodicals of the day. These include *The American Journal of Insanity, The Alienist and Neurologist, The Journal of Mental Science, The Journal of Nervous and Mental Diseases,* and *Mind.* As well, it is essential to become acquainted with several crucial monographs by prominent Victorian biomedical theorists. Chief among these are W.B. Carpenter's *Principle of Human Physiology,* American edition (Philadelphia: Blanchard & Lea, 1855), and *Principles of Mental Physiology* (New York: Appleton, 1874); Alexander Bain, *The Emotions and The Will,* 3rd edition, (London: Longmans, Green, 1880) and *The Senses and the Intellect,* 3rd edition (London: Longmans, Green, 1868); J.C. Bucknill and Daniel H. Tuke, *A Manual of Psychological Medicine* (Philadelphia: Blanchard and Lea, 1858); and Henry Maudsley, *The Pathology of Mind* (London: Macmillan, 1879).

Introduction

In the distant heyday of Victorian biography it was fashionable to preface the subject's name in the title with the phrase "the life and times." Since the eventual consequence of these eulogistic and didactic volumes was to consign biography to the fringe of professional historical writing, it would be imprudent to employ such a designation for the present work. But the phrase is, nonetheless, an apt characterization for the content of this study: It is an account of an individual medical life set within the context of its professional times. Unfortunately most social historians, particularly in fields such as the history of science, have been relatively reticent in adopting such methodology. For medical historians this reluctance is in part a reaction against what has been styled the *great-doctors approach*.[1] As a result, major figures of nineteenth-century American psychiatry–John P. Gray, Pliny Earle, Isaac Ray–and their counterparts in England–James C. Pritchard, John Conolly, Daniel H. Tuke, Henry Maudsley–are without twentieth-century biographers.[2] Yet as a reviewer observed in reference to a study of René Villerme and French sanitary theory, it is possible for an author to succeed in "depicting the life of his hero as a social event."[3] This, in essence, is the methodological goal of the social historian who turns to biography.

In the present study, the career of Richard M. Bucke, a Canadian alienist, provides the superstructure for an analysis of major themes in late nineteenth-century Anglo-American psychiatry. Born in Great Britain in 1837, educated at McGill University and, later, in London and Paris, he practiced in Canada, traveled often to England, and sought his professional peers among American alienists. Following his appointment to an asylum superintendency in 1876 he became intimately familiar with the contemporary English-language literature on insanity and published a number of papers, particularly in the *American Journal of Insanity,* and two books of relevance to psychiatry, *Man's Moral Nature* (1879) and *Cosmic Consciousness* (1901). He numbered among his many medical acquaintances William Osler and S. Weir Mitchell in the United States and Benjamin Ward Richardson and Sir William Jenner in Great Britain, and was visited at his institution by prominent alienists from both countries, including Henry Hurd and Daniel H. Tuke. Symbolic of his trans-Atlantic professional identity, he was elected president of the British Medical Association's Psychological Section in 1897 and of the American Medico–Psychological Association the following year. He died, accidentally, in 1902.[4]

In many important respects, it will be argued, Bucke was a physician who typified a generation of Victorian psychiatrists. A fascinating and often eccentric individual, he was well known to both his medical contemporaries and later historians as much for his unorthodox literary opinions – specifically, his championship of Walt Whitman[5] and his role in the Bacon–Shakespeare debate – or for his seeming mysticism[6] as for his psychiatric theorizing.[7] Yet it must be admitted that he was in no sense a figure of towering stature or authority in his discipline. Indeed, what is striking about Bucke the alienist was, not his originality, but his very lack of it. Through his mind, a great, open-meshed colander, poured the medical literature of his day. Some major concepts and many minor intellectual fragments were caught, to reappear, albeit with an idiosyncratic twist, in both his published work and in his asylum practice. If, however, he was representative of the broad outlines of late nineteenth-century biology and medical psychology, at times he revealed rather marked departures from orthodoxy. On these occasions he may be portrayed by the historian as a foil: By contrasting his attitudes to those of his contemporaries, or studying their reaction to his views, it is possible to gain an understanding less of Bucke himself than of the contemporaneous psychiatric consensus. For example, though much of Bucke's asylum therapy was typical of his generation of alienists, his excursion into gynecological surgery as a form of psychotherapy was highly idiosyncratic and provoked a revealing reaction on the part of his professional contemporaries. In effect, Bucke's departures from typicality are as useful for studying the wider context of

Anglo-American psychiatry as are those areas in which he evinced a steadfast orthodoxy.

With Bucke as the central character, the following study describes the nature and genesis of late nineteenth-century psychiatry. Psychiatric theory and practice were, in the first instance, the product of individual men, physicians who brought with them to the asylum ideas colored by the personal and medical environment in which they were nurtured.[8] Chapter 1 of this study, largely narrative, describes Bucke's background and the process by which he, like many of his contemporaries, acquired his medical mindset. Yet the practice of institutional psychiatry was by no means a direct reflection of medical doctrines, for the asylums in which alienists found themselves assumed an autonomous character often quite at odds with the assumptions of their creators.[9] The process by which Bucke's institution fashioned its own complex identity is described in Chapter 2.

Neither individual physicians nor their institutions existed, of course, in a social vacuum. The distinction between psychiatric ideas and social theory becomes increasingly indistinct and artificial as the assumptions underlying medical rhetoric are explored.[10] In Bucke's case his physiology was the biological expression of positivism, while his theory of psychopathology was a medical statement of contemporaneous beliefs concerning poverty and social degeneration. These themes are discussed in Chapters 3 and 4. Finally, psychiatrists as a group had professional ambitions which were translated into specific therapeutic strategies calculated to enhance such aspirations. This topic is the focus of Chapter 5.

Taken together, then, individual physicians, institutional character, dominant social values, and explicit professional goals combined to determine the nature of late-Victorian psychiatry. To untangle the complex interaction of these various elements is the purpose of the following study.

1

The topography of a Victorian medical life

Richard Maurice Bucke grew to professional maturity in a period of turbulence for Anglo-American medicine. Within a year of his entry into medical school, Rudolph Virchow had challenged two millenia of humoralism with his treatise on cellular pathology, while Charles Darwin's description of evolution permanently redirected the biological sciences. Shortly after Bucke's graduation, the work of Pasteur began the process of explaining infectious diseases, a process Koch's classic study of anthrax significantly enhanced in the year Bucke received his asylum appointment. Though cures were still elusive, the heroic therapeutics popular before midcentury – bleeding, purging, and dosing with toxic quantities of pharmaceuticals – were disappearing by the time Bucke reached McGill, replaced, instead, by an emphasis on accurate physical diagnosis and conservative, symptomatic therapy. This new therapeutic restraint, together with antiseptic surgery, allowed hospitals to shed their traditional charnel-house image. Often indistinguishable from the almshouse in the early years of the century, hospitals had become, by the 1870s attractive to a more affluent middle-class patient. Within these institutions physicians, buoyed less by effective new therapeutics than by the authority of their newly acquired, value-transcendent vocabulary of science, gained in economic status and social power. New licensing laws, uniform educational standards, and a proliferation of medical journals and societies attested to the profession's increasingly homogeneous and esoteric character. It was within this evolving professional environment that Bucke absorbed his basic assumptions as to the potential and the limitations of clinical medicine. His career was to be shaped by precisely those forces that would so dramatically alter the practice and structure of Anglo-American medicine during the Victorian period.

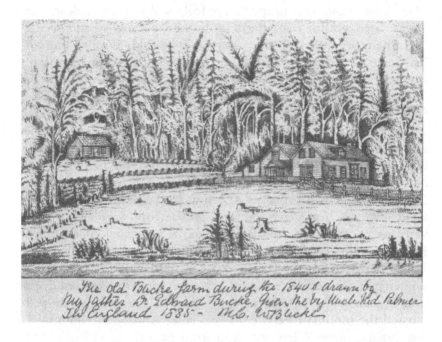

Figure 1. The Bucke family farm near London, Ontario, c. 1840.
Source: R. M. Bucke Collection, University of Western Ontario.

Bucke was born in England in 1837, the son of a Church of
England cleric and the great-great-grandson of Prime Minister
Sir Robert Walpole. The following year the family, including
seven of an eventual ten children, emigrated to upper Canada,
then in the turbulent aftermath of rebellion. They settled at
Creek Farm (Figure 1) near the future site of the London Asylum
and Bucke seems to have led an idyllic rural existence uninter-
rupted by the drudgery of formal schooling.[1] Instead, turned
loose in his father's immense library, he read Marryat's novels,
Scott's poems, and, significantly, Robert Chamber's *Vestiges of
the Natural History of Creation* (1845).[2] Even at this early stage, he
seems to have developed a deep interest in the metaphysical questions that would dominate his adult life. Though he claimed
never to have accepted Christian doctrines of eternal punishment,
a vengeful God, or a divine afterlife, he "dwelt on these and
similar topics far more than anyone would suppose."[3] But death
intruded on his adolescent world, leaving him an orphan by

1854. The events that immediately followed remain unclear, but Bucke later recalled that affairs "at home went badly" and his life "became more unhappy than can readily be told." Feeling himself "ill-treated," he resolved to leave "home and live or die as might happen." For the next three years he wandered the American West, working at first in Ohio as a gardener, a railway man, and a farm laborer, and later cutting staves in the swamps of Louisiana and plying the Mississippi as a riverboat deckhand.[4] In 1856 he moved west from Missouri, and six months later, after a narrow brush with Indian raiders, arrived on the eastern slope of the Sierra Nevadas. Finding it was too late in the year to reach California, Bucke turned his hand to prospecting in the small settlement of Gold Canyon. Among his fellow prospectors were two young veterans of the California gold fields, Allen and Hosea Grosh. Following the latter's death from blood poisoning, Allen and Bucke departed for the Pacific coast in the fall of 1857. An early winter met the two adventurers, trapping them in five-foot drifts near Squaw Valley. After an epic struggle, the unfortunate pair crossed the mountains and collapsed at an isolated mining camp. Twelve days later Allen was dead from exposure and Bucke had lost all of one frostbitten foot and part of the other.[5]

Bucke returned to Canada in 1858, as he later phrased it, "a cripple, a wreck"[6] and, with no clear motive other than the example of two older brothers, used an inheritance to enroll in medicine at McGill University.[7] It was a fortunate choice, for the quality of the school was then rivaled on the American continent only by Philadelphia.[8] From the beginning in 1822, the school offered two features unique in North America. First, its proprietors, following the example of Edinburgh where they had all taken a portion of their own training, insisted that students be given full freedom of the wards at the Montreal General Hospital. Secondly, at a time when most American shcools required attendance for two four-month sessions, McGill demanded four six-month terms.[9] To qualify for a degree, students were required to attend lectures in botany and zoology, demonstrate competence in classics, give proof of twelve months' attendance at the hospital, and submit a thesis. In medical subjects, candidates were examined in anatomy, chemistry, *materia medica* and pharmacology, and the institutes of medicine, a discipline comprised of histology, physiology, general pathology, and general therapeutics. Final exami-

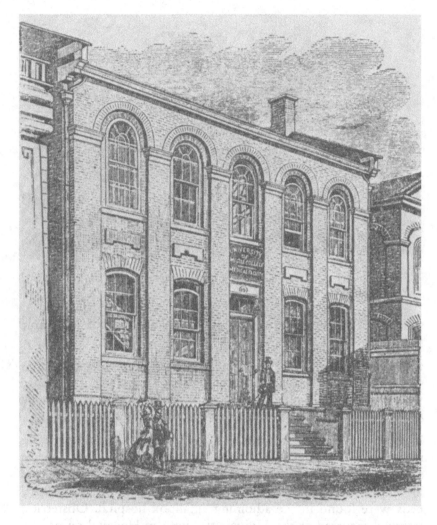

Figure 2. Medical Faculty, McGill University, c. 1858. Source: *Journal of Education for Lower Canada,* vol. 2, no. 4, April 1858, p. 50.

nations, entirely oral, in the practice of medicine, surgery, midwifery, and medical jurisprudence completed the requirements.[10] To Maurice Bucke in 1858, with no previous formal schooling to swell his confidence, the prospect of successfully clearing these academic hurdles must have seemed elusive.

The medical faculty's quarters (Figure 2) in which Bucke

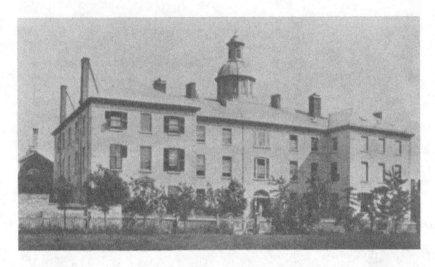

Figure 3. Montreal General Hospital, 1850s. Source: Montreal General Hospital.

studied had opened in 1851. A graduate later recalled its simple facilities:

On entering the old Côté Street Building the museum was on the right side of the passage and the library on the left. At the end of the passage was a large lecture room. Upstairs the whole front was the dissecting room, and there was another large lecture room in the rear.[11]

Fortunately, the faculty was provided with additional teaching space at the Montreal General Hospital (Figure 3) which, in the 1860s, could accommodate 150 patients in "many ill-lighted and ill-ventilated rooms" in the main building, and supplementary beds were found in the adjoining smallpox hospital. Obstetrical training occurred at the University Lying-in Hospital on nearby Urbain Street, an enterprise founded by the wives of the medical professors to serve working-class patients. When Osler arrived at the Montreal General eight years after Bucke had graduated, he found it "an old coccus- and rat-ridden building" redeemed by its "two valuable assets for the student – much acute disease and a group of keen teachers." Surgical and medical services were not separated, he recalled, and students encountered pneumonia, phthisis, sepsis, and dysentery while serving as dressers or clerks.[12] Other common conditions of the period included delir-

ium tremens, frostbite, and periodic epidemics of cholera, typhus, typhoid, and smallpox. These diseases were treated with
leeches, blisters, and prescriptions "of the blunderbuss variety, in
the hope that something would hit the mark." Among the pharmaceuticals in common use were digitalis, potassium iodide,
silver nitrate, Dover's powders, *lotio rubra,* morphine, quinine,
and an enormous volume of alcohol. Surgery was resorted to
with reluctance. In the late 1860s both the wooden floor of the
operating room and the operating table itself were "blood-
stained and reeking with odours," a condition apparently shared
by the surgical instruments and the surgeon's ' "old frock coat"
as well. The "abdomen was never opened except accidently" and
the few standard procedures consisted largely of ligature of arter-
ies, extirpation of tumors, the removal of bladder stones, and
amputations. In this pre-Listerian period, one Montreal student
recalled, "I do not think I ever saw a case of amputation of the
thigh recover," while strangulated hernia "resulted usually in
fatality."[13] Faced with the often-disappointing results of "blunderbuss" medicine and a frightening surgical mortality, the
medical staff were at pains to preserve their students from complete surrender to the rising tides of therapeutic nihilism.[14]

During the years Bucke spent at McGill, the school had yet to
establish a sequential curriculum. Students were expected to attend each course in primary and clinical subjects, exluding medical
jurisprudence, for two sessions, supplemented in the final year by
formal clinical work at the hospital. Lectures began at nine each
morning, finishing at eight in the evening, and were followed by
two hours of anatomical dissection (Figure 4).[15] Though the lectures in basic science appear to have been dull recitations from
textbooks, unaccompanied by laboratory work,[16] clinical instruction, particularly from Osler's future mentor, R. Palmer
Howard, was substantially more inspired.[17] Bucke's clinical notes
that have survived reveal little speculation on causation, but a
great deal of emphasis on the natural history of certain illnesses
and on physical diagnosis. In the case of phthisis, he noted in detail
the progressive stages of the disease, the changing signs elicited by
auscultation and percussion, and the microscopic appearance of
the sputum. "Never," he reminded himself, "make a diagnosis
from the first examination." These notes and those on smallpox,
chronic bronchitis, or emphysema discouraged aggressive ther-

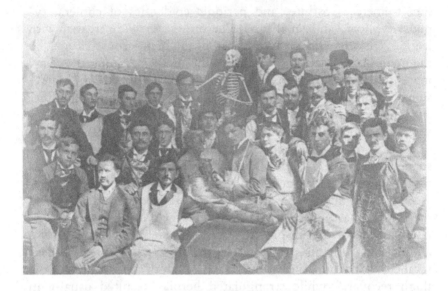

Figure 4. Anatomy class, n.d.; likely McGill University, c. 1860.
Source: R. M. Bucke Collection, University of Western Ontario.

apy, adopting instead the maxim: "Watch case and treat symptoms as they arise." His instruction in the examination of the
patient stressed the importance of accurate observation and the
detection of subtle clinical signs. In taking a medical history and
a review of systems, Professor MacCallum advised the clinical
novice to "let the patient give it in his own words" and his pupils
were warned, too, against the all-too-common fallacy of dismiss-
ing common afflictions as "scarcely worth attention," in preference to cases of "internal aneurism, incurable heart affliction, or
some form of malignant disease."[18] The medical education Bucke
received at McGill, then, was designed primarily to enable the
physician to diagnose disease accurately, to treat its symptomatic
manifestations appropriately, and to offer the patient a realistic
prognosis. Neither surgery nor medicine in this period offered
routine promise of curative intervention, a perspective which
was to be reflected in Bucke's subsequent career as a physician.

Shortly after graduating in 1862 with several academic prizes in
hand, Bucke departed for postgraduate studies in London.
Among the city's eleven medical schools pride of place rested
with the two new institutions affiliated with the University of

London: University College and King's College, and their re-
spective hospitals.[19] It was to these that Bucke was attracted,
though he attended clinics at smaller specialty institutions as
well. While both had been in existence barely three decades, they
could lay claim to impressive innovations. It was at University
College Hospital that Robert Liston introduced anesthesia to
British surgery in 1846, while King's, largely at the instigation of
the physiologist and surgeon Robert Bentley Todd, became in
1856 the first hospital in the country to staff its wards with fully
trained nurses.[20] These institutions numbered among their staff
many of the most prominent English physicians of the period.
William Sharpey, whose lectures Bucke attended, was Professor
of Anatomy and Physiology at University College. Though he
produced scant original work, he was an outstanding teacher and
his lectures, antivitalist and sympathetic to Darwinian theory,
would clearly have appealed to Bucke.[21] William Fergusson at
King's College was perhaps the leading London surgeon of his
day, unmatched, it was said, in the rapidity and precision of his
technique. The speed of his style derived from his training in the
pre-anesthetic period and to the end of his career he repaired cleft
palates without the use of such agents.[22] At University College
Hospital the professor of clinical surgery was Richard Quain, a
cautious surgeon noted for his publications on vascular and rectal
operations. Bucke observed his work and met Quain socially,
likely finding an affinity with his host's interest in English literature. Even more congenial, perhaps, was Quain's colleague, Sir
Henry Thompson, whose surgery Bucke also observed. His primary interest was urology and he numbered a substantial assort-
ment of European royalty among his satisfied patients. Beyond
his medical works, he wrote several novels and his paintings
were exhibited at the Royal Academy. His greatest fame derived
from his role in founding the controversial Cremation Society of
England in 1874 and from his subsequent publication of a pan-
theistic philosophy, similar to that of his friends Tyndall, Huxley, and Spencer, in 1902.[23] Though Bucke was never to practice
surgery himself, he absorbed, while in England, a deep respect
for the accomplishments and potential of that specialty.

Among the internists with whom Bucke studied, the most
prominent was Sir William Jenner who held the chair in medicine
at University College and was later to become Physician Extra-

ordinary to Queen Victoria. He was known for his clinical–
pathological differentiation of typhus and typhoid, which confirmed the conclusions of Pierre Louis and W. W. Gerhard, and
for his monograph on diphtheria. Jenner's lectures were lucid
presentations, devoid of speculation, and frequently emphasizing
sanitary prevention as preferable to curative intervention. He was
an exacting bedside teacher, requiring precision of both style and
substance in cases presented by his students. Having excelled in
case notes at McGill, Bucke may have made a sound impression
on Jenner; certainly, the professor impressed Bucke. He met Jenner socially through friends and requested his opinion on a disorder that troubled one of his brothers. Later he consulted him
concerning his own abdominal ailments and sought his testimonial in support of his application for an asylum position.[24] He
also attended lectures by two of Jenner's junior colleagues.
Thomas Hillier gave instruction on diseases of the skin and Russell Reynolds specialized in neurological disorders. The latter had
assumed the practice of the celebrated neurologist Marshall Hall
upon his retirement, and he himself went on to publish a number
of papers on vertigo, epilepsy, and insanity. He was best known
as editor of *A System of Medicine,* published in five volumes between 1866 and 1879 and containing contributions by a number
of noted English physicians. Each volume of this work Bucke
eagerly acquired as it was published and appeared, in his practice,
to rely on its authority.[25]

Not all of Bucke's medical influences were limited to King's or
University College Hospitals. He attended clinics at the Royal
London Ophthalmic Hospital (Moorfields), where a likely contact was Jonathan Hutchinson, a surgeon–dermatologist whose
wide range of medical interests led Osler to describe him as "the
last of the polymaths."[26] His textbook on syphilitic diseases of
the ear and eye Bucke certainly read while in London.[27] In his
personal life, Hutchinson rejected the Christian concept of afterlife, borrowing instead from Darwin to forge his own evolutionary philosophy, which he termed *Terralism.* Like many of his
contemporaries he believed the growth in human knowledge was
directly transmissible to offspring, a transmission that guaranteed
the ultimate elevation of the human race to a higher plane of
existence. This concept bore a marked resemblance to that which
would become the thesis of Bucke's study of *cosmic consciousness.*

Even if Bucke did not discuss these philosophical ideas with Hutchinson, the surgeon may have contributed significantly to the development of his thought in two other areas. First, during the late 1850s, Hutchinson had worked with Spencer Wells to revive the controversial operation ovariotomy, a procedure that Bucke would endorse for the surgical treatment of insane women thirty years later. Second, in 1859 Hutchinson persuaded Hughlings Jackson, subsequently to become Britain's most noted late nineteenth-century neurologist, not to abandon medicine for a career in philosophy. For the next four years Jackson lived with Hutchinson and through his influence secured a clinical assistantship at Moorfields.[28] It is possible that Bucke may have encountered Jackson there and found that they shared a common interest in both philosophy and agnosticism. Whether such a meeting occurred is not recorded in Bucke's diary, but his later views on insanity as a form of nervous devolution reveal similarities to theories published by Jackson during the 1870s. Had they met, Bucke might later have felt an affinity for the work of a former Moorfields acquaintance.

The clinician who seems to have had the most direct influence on Bucke was Sir Benjamin Ward Richardson, physician to several London hospitals, Dean of St. George's School of Medicine, and a close acquaintance of Bucke's friend, Harry Forman. Though only nine years Bucke's senior, he was already well known for his clinical work on blood transfusions, his description of the cardiovascular effects of amyl nitrate, and his discovery of a number of local and general anesthetics. He was also a minor literary figure who had published a novel and belonged to "Our Club" which included as members the author, William Thackeray, and the founder of *Punch*, Mark Lemon. His major contribution to medical literature was in the field of public health and preventive medicine. With his friends William Farr and Sir Edwin Chadwick, he emphasized the importance of sanitary legislation and accurate health statistics as the key to social improvement. He never appears to have conceded the validity of germ theory, remaining convinced throughout his life that health was most closely related to life style and that disease – tuberculosis, for example – was most effectively treated with sound diet, moderate exercise, and fresh air. It was this perspective that informed his well-publicized, though unpopular, condemnation of the medical and social use of alcohol. Received with much greater enthusiasm was his 1875 address, "Hygeia: A City of Health," in which he envisaged a utopian metropolis from which sanitary reforms had all but banished disease. It was a theme to which he returned in his *Diseases of Modern Life* (1876), a popular commentary on the relationship between mental and physical pathology and the excesses of Victorian existence, similar in tone to the publications of the American neurologist, George M. Beard.[29] It is clear that Richardson's attitude toward therapeutics, especially alcohol, influenced Bucke's own approach to treatment. Harry Forman kept him informed of Richardson's publications and relayed replies to inquiries from Bucke on medical topics. Bucke sent him a copy of his first paper on the nervous system, and, when applying for his asylum position, he received "a very handsome testimonial from Dr. Richardson."[30] Of the various physicians he encountered in England, then, it would seem that Richardson exerted the most enduring influence.

Maurice Bucke's exposure to English medicine was followed by four months in Paris. Upon arrival he attended a lecture on fractures of the femur at the Ecole de Médicine, but discovered with frustration, "I understood scarcely a word, certainly I did not catch a single idea." He plunged into French literature, intending to master the language by that summer. A month later he felt his reading "goes on as easy as an old shoe" and he resolved "to make a start" on daily attendance at the hospital. He listened to lectures by Armand Trousseau and he read his textbook, *Clinique Médicale de l'Hôtel Dieu* (1861), in neither case finding the language difficult. At the Hôpital des Enfants Malades he saw "A great many fine cases – Pott's curvature, deformities from rickets," and his ever-roving eye caught sight of a clinical phenomenon as yet unknown in Canada, "a lady student . . . young – but not bad looking." At La Charité he made ward rounds with Joseph Beau, known best as an authority on cardiopulmonary disorders, and saw "a lot of women treated for ulceration, inflammation, etc., of the *os uteri*."[31] Paris, it seemed, offered Bucke the wide range of clinical experience to which the privileged elite among his generation of North American medical graduates were attracted. Before 1820, ambitious students might have gone to Edinburgh, while later in the century, Germany exerted the dominant attraction. At midcentury, however, American graduates made their way to Paris where admission to the hospital wards, lecture theaters, and outpatient clinics was free and additional private tutelage was to be had for modest fees. In the forty years following 1820, 677 American graduates studied in Paris, more than at any other single location abroad.[32] This situation would change, with an estimated 15,000 Americans studying in German universities between 1870 and 1914, but at midcentury foreign training for a North American graduate remained a relatively unique and prestigious accomplishment.[33]

In France the early nineteenth century had produced a generation of unique and talented teachers, particularly Pierre Jean-George Cabanis, Xavier Bichat, and Philippe Pinel. These men were the forerunners of what came to be called the *Paris Clinical School,* a style of medicine represented by the work of René Laennec, celebrated as the inventor of the stethoscope, and Pierre Louis, best known for his statistical approach to clinical problems. The accomplishments of this school were widely reported in North American medical journals, recounted in observations by "medical tourists," and made available through translated editions of significant works. Though adopting diverse and often contradictory perspectives, the members of the Paris School appeared to agree on a fundamental clinical philosophy. It was an approach that stressed the necessity of correlating clinical signs and symptoms with pathological findings at autopsy, as well as the importance of collecting a large series of such cases before announcing a conclusion as to the nature of a particular disease. This perspective left no room for etiological speculation and was coupled with a marked therapeutic skepticism, that is, a preference for an expectant approach to therapy, a predilection for local rather than generalized treatment, and a tendency to avoid drugs in favor of diet, bathing, and exercise. Microscopy, animal experimentation, and laboratory chemistry played no role in this essentially clinical approach to medicine.[34] In the first half of the nineteenth century, it was a philosophy that appeared innovative and refreshing to postgraduate students wearied of groundless theories and therapeutics based on little but tradition.

The "last of the great classic clinicians" and "the most eloquent and elegant of Paris professors" was Armand Trousseau, the professor whose lectures and text Bucke chose to study. A classicist and teacher of rhetoric before becoming a physician, Trousseau held the chair in clinical medicine at Hôtel Dieu and was a

pioneer in introducing tracheotomy, thoracentesis, and intuba-
tion to Parisian medicine. Despite these accomplishments and his
polished lecture style, he did not attract many American students, though among French students he was famous for his
treatise on therapeutics published in 1836. He was, in general, an
eclectic with a marked streak of skepticism, recommending intervention only when absolutely necessary and proclaiming his faith
in the healing power of nature. He did suggest the use of drugs
but was an exponent of local treatment, such as the use of tracheotomy in diphtheria, whenever possible. He was willing to acknowledge the importance of the psychological manifestations of
diseases such as hyperthyroidism, angina pectoris, and asthma,
including as evidence, in the case of the latter, his own experiences. Finally, he was convinced that experimental physiology
and biochemistry had little to contribute to clinical medicine, a
viewpoint illustrated by his opposition to Paul Broca's early theories on the cerebral localization of the speech center.[35] Bucke's
own conservative approach to therapeutics and his lack of enthusiasm for experimental medicine were doubtless in part a reflection of his exposure to Trousseau and the Paris School.

In the early summer of 1863 Bucke found himself suffering
from an attack of "ague." A month later, "thin as blazes" and in
a "state of semi-vitality," he concluded that his fever "must have
been typhoid." Physically weakened, he soon discovered that his
finances were vitiated as well, forcing him to abandon his plans
to study in Berlin. He returned to England for several months
and, after receiving news of the illness of his brother, Dr. Edward Bucke of Sarnia, sailed for Canada on the day before
Christmas, 1863. On arrival, he was greeted with the news of his
brother's demise and soon after took over his medical practice.[36]
Though he interrupted his professional activities to spend almost
a year in California serving, in return for a substantial retainer, as
a witness in the Grosh family's claim to a share in the Comstock
silver lode, he returned to Sarnia in 1865.[37] Several months later
he married Jessie Gurd, whom he had courted intermittently
since beginning his medical studies, and settled down to the serious business of building a medical career (Figure 5).[38]

It was an auspicious time to enter the province's medical profession. Physicians in Ontario during the 1860s were in fact, in a
transitional phase, moving from a loose collection of diversely

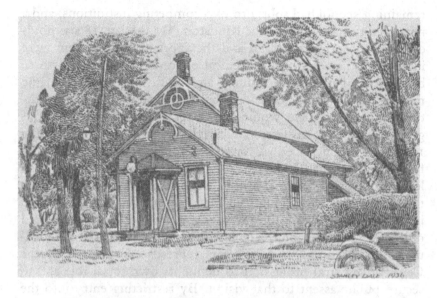

Figure 5. Office occupied by R. M. Bucke's medical practice in Sarnia, Ontario, during the 1860s (sketched in 1936). Source: R. M. Bucke Collection, University of Western Ontario.

qualified individuals toward a body of practitioners of uniform training and homogeneous medical opinions. In the year Bucke opened his office a new medical act attempted to define this change in status. It entrusted registration to a central medical body empowered both to determine the content of the curriculum in the province's medical schools and to accord the protection of the law (a protection which included, for example, the right to sue for fees) only to duly licensed physicians. Certainly, many "irregulars" continued to practice, and both homeopathic and eclectic practitioners were still recognized as legitimate professional variants under earlier legislation. But the 1865 act served as a necessary prelude to another bill four years later which permanently established the Ontario College of Physicians and Surgeons and required that all registrants pass a uniform licensing exam.[39] That provision for an independent examination was necessary was attested to by the diverse forms and uneven quality of medical training available within the province. In 1853, for example, Ontario's three medical schools were all to be found in Toronto. Three years later two of these no longer existed, the remaining school had split into two competing institutions, and a new faculty had appeared at Kingston. By the late 1860s, however, the proprietary school and the apprenticeship system were increasingly anachronistic. Medical education was henceforth to be a form of university training and, with the exception of the medical faculty at Victoria University in Cobourg, those institutions existing in 1870 would prove to be permanent.[40] To this groundwork for professional development established in the 1860s was soon added a variety of medical societies, ranging from the Canadian Medical Association, established in 1867, to local groups such as the Toronto Medical Society, revived under that name in 1878. Though no medical journals were published in the province during the 1860s, seven new periodicals appeared during the next decade.[41] The institutional and legislative innovations that occurred in these years represented attempts by the Canadian medical profession to define its own social role and to secure public assent to that vision. By restricting entry into the profession to those individuals possessed of orthodox training, physicians purported to offer the public a comforting guarantee of predictable standards and methods of practice. In return, they demanded and received the right to professional self-government and a monopoly on the provision of health care.[42] If this exchange became the accepted norm by the twentieth century, it was clearly a novelty in the 1860s.

Maurice Bucke began his medical practice in a period in which the social position of physicians, if not immediately enhanced, was gradually clarified and institutionalized. But though status changed in these years, the content and style of daily practice remained remarkably constant.[43] Hospital practice was unknown outside the largest cities and even there problems arose. The Toronto General Hospital, for example, was portrayed in the local press of the 1850s as little more than a charnel house and in 1867 was forced to close for almost a year due to lack of financial support. Given the popular aversion to hospitals, such surgery as was done during the 1860s was usually performed in the patient's home, with the anesthetic often administered by a family member. The operations attempted were generally either relatively minor or necessitated by trauma. In the period preceding Listerian antisepsis, undertaking a major procedure such as opening the abdomen or chest almost always resulted in a fatal infection.

In fact, as one Toronto graduate of 1871 recalled, to that date "there was not, so far as I know, one abdomen opened in the Toronto General Hospital."[44]

Pharmaceutical intervention was equally limited in efficacy though it was, in view of the obvious physiological alterations induced by many drugs, often presumed by patients to possess curative value. Quinine helped to deal with the malaria endemic to the Great Lakes basin during the nineteenth century and vaccination prevented the spread of smallpox. A variety of emetics and cathartics, some opium, and vast quantities of alcohol were frequently employed, alone or in combinations, to treat a variety of common complaints.[45] The effect of such treatment in the epidemics of cholera which plagued Ontario from 1832 to 1871, as well as in other significant epidemics of typhus, typhoid, scarlet fever, and measles, was at best symptomatic. In the case of "the white plague," tuberculosis, the leading cause of adult death in this period, even the treatment of symptoms was difficult and of transient value.[46] A steady supply of patients, nonetheless, seem to have filled the offices of general practitioners or, almost as frequently, to have sought consultations in their own homes. The outcome in serious cases of the latter type may have been as dependent on adequate transportation and communication links as on the range of pharmaceuticals available.[47] In addition to the symptomatic treatment that the physicians dispensed, patients derived a sense of security from hearing a diagnostic label applied to their infirmities and had their apprehensions confirmed or denied when given a considered prognosis. To many patients, perhaps 70%, this solace was of sufficient value to prompt them to pay their doctor, whether in kind or in cash.[48] The nature of midcentury general practice, it would seem, was readily compatible with the conservative medical philosophy Maurice Bucke had acquired in London and Paris. His approach to his practice did not depart significantly from that of his professional contemporaries.

The cases Bucke encountered differed little from those seen by general practitioners well into the twentieth century, though the relative proportions of each type may have varied somewhat. For example, acute infections were slightly more common, while degenerative diseases were less so.[49] Though his diagnoses ranged from goiter to "sluggish liver," gastrointestinal complaints formed the largest single category, followed closely by respiratory disease.[50] Gynecological disorders, usually termed *leukorrhea,* suggesting an undifferentiated vaginal discharge, and minor neurological conditions, particularly *hemicrania* or migraine headache, were also frequently encountered. Midwifery occupied some of his time, though he disliked the erratic hours. On occasion he administered an anesthetic while another surgeon performed the operation, and he made conscientious home visits to patients recuperating from a procedure. He seems to have maintained a skeptical attitude toward some widely prescribed medicines, commenting, for example, on another physician's patient who "does not get well very fast after her typhoid fever and calomel."[51] Nor was he prepared to accept uncritically new theories of disease, observing of the suggestion that tuberculosis originated in follicular pharyngitis, "I do not think the theory amounts to shucks." Similarly, of the hyperbaric chamber he saw in Toronto, a "new invention for curing all disorders," he felt "there is likely something in the affair but [I] am afraid this will not be managed so that we shall find out what." In his own practice he seemed to rely on few diagnostic aids though he did possess a microscope, with which he examined skin cancers. Psychiatric disorders played a minor and unwelcome role in his practice. He recorded a single case of suicide in his diary and clearly disliked the court testimony required of him "on a beastly case of insanity." Less severe forms of emotional stress, however, were common and he commented, "I have witnessed sentiment enough to make half a dozen ordinary three vol. novels."[52] Maurice Bucke's practice, then, was a not untypical mixture of coughs and abdominal upsets, a little midwifery and surgery, and a dash of madness.[53]

Whatever the nature of his cases, Bucke's days were more than full. His medical ledger suggests that he saw an average of ten patients a day, including weekends, either at his office or in their homes. He was also engaged to provide medical services on behalf of the inhabitants of the nearby Indian reservation. Though his daily volume of patients represented a small number of consultations by later standards, it meant, as Bucke explained to Harry Forman, "I work on an average from 12 to 14 hours a day." As his practice grew, so did the demands made on his time, particularly as calls often involved traveling substantial distances by boat or horseback. On one occasion Bucke complained bitterly, "I have had one full night's sleep in the last seven nights, three of these nights I did not have my clothes off at all."[54] In return for his efforts, over the first four years in practice, he billed $16,462.46 and received $10,703.51, a collection rate of 65%. As he observed to Forman, "this is not perhaps a great deal of money . . . but it is a great deal to make in a small town and country practice." He later admitted, however, that he found himself "infernally hard up a good part of the time," largely because he had spent $2,500 on a lot and house for his growing family. It was to prove a necessary expenditure since, though his first child, born in 1866, died at ten months, two other children followed by 1870 and five more appeared over the next decade.[55] In fact, despite the limitations imposed on his time by the demands of practice, Bucke seems to have become a model family man. He confided his deep affection for his children to Alfred Forman, all but abandoned the use of alcohol and tobacco, and though "disgusted" at himself, periodically agreed to attend church with Jessie. Yet for all the attractions of home or the frantic pace of practice, it was an existence with which Bucke remained vaguely discontent. As he phrased it in his diary, "My life . . . now that I am fairly married and settled down to work is so monotonous that what is said for one day answers for every other day."[56]

The familiar routine, however, was not to last. For two months in the fall of 1870 Bucke wrestled with dysentery and, after a recuperation in England, found it necessary to confine his medical work to the town of Sarnia and limit his night calls to established patients. Several months later his health was still "not first class" which he attributed to "the villanous malaria here." Apparently another convalescent trip was taken to England in the spring of 1872, during which Bucke consulted Sir William Jenner and received a report "on the whole satisfactory."[57] It was during this trip that Bucke underwent a unique and profound experience, an event which, in retrospect, is made comprehensible only through an appreciation of certain aspects of his personality. During a fourteen-year period a psychological affliction appeared sporadically and in various guises in his diaries: He was subject to periodic attacks of what twentieth-century practitioners would refer to as acute anxiety. On one occasion the episode seems to have been little more than a free-floating sense of foreboding, while on another it was more substantial. "[I] had in the middle of the night," he wrote in 1864, "one of my old attacks – sort of nightmare – have not had one before for about 15 years." Whether these attacks provided part of Bucke's motive in consulting Sir William Jenner is unclear, but he seems to have discussed his condition while there with his uncle. "I cannot contemplate anything so horrible as your breaking down," Biggs Andrews wrote to his nephew, "you must not *be too anxious*." Despite this injunction the problem persisted and two years later he described "a violent attack of nervous depression from Dyspepsia." Indeed, periods of acute anxiety or panic attacks seem to have been a recurrent problem for Bucke.[58]

Insight into the precise character of these episodes may be gained from a paper that Bucke read at a meeting of American asylum superintendents in 1877. He discussed, in passing, the "pathological conditions of the stomach which produce terror and low spirits." To illustrate his point he described an attack of "nervous dyspepsia" which was "taken word for word from the account given to the present writer by the actual sufferer, who is himself a highly intellectual medical man." Indeed, he elaborated, the description "refers to one particular attack, which was witnessed by the writer." In fact, interpreted in light of his diaries, it is clear that Bucke was indulging in an autobiographical exercise. He described the attack in the following terms:

A man is suffering from what we call nervous dyspepsia. Some day, we will suppose in the middle of the afternoon, without any warning or visible cause, one of these attacks of terror come on. The first thing the man feels is a great but vague discomfort. Then he notices that his heart is beating much too violently. At the same time shocks or flashes as of electrical discharges so violent as to be almost painful, and accompanied by a feeling of extreme distress, pass one after another through his body and limbs. Then in a few minutes he falls into a condition of the most intense fear. He is not afraid of anything; he is simply afraid. His mind is perfectly clear. He looks for a cause for his wretched condition, but sees none. Presently his terror is such that he trembles violently, and utters low moans; his body is damp with perspiration; his mouth is perfectly dry; and at this stage there are no tears in his eyes, though his suffering is intense. When the climax of the attack is reached and passed, there is copious flow of tears, or else a mental condition in which the person weeps upon the least provocation. At this stage a large quantity of pale urine is passed. Then the heart's action becomes again normal, and the attack passes off.

Only after consulting "a couple of the best alienists on the continent" in 1878, did his "series of nervous attacks" seem to abate.[59]

When Bucke visited England in 1872 he experienced an attack of quite a different nature but one which may have been related to his labile emotions and history of anxiety states. Almost thirty years later he published an account of that episode, which William James considered a classic example of mystical illumination.[60] According to Bucke, speaking in the third person:

It was in the early spring at the beginning of his thirty-sixth year. He and two friends had spent the evening reading Wordsworth, Shelley, Keats, Browning, and especially Whitman. They parted at midnight, and he had a long drive in a hansom (it was in an English city). His mind deeply under the influence of the ideas, images and emotions called up by the reading and talk of the evening, was calm and peaceful. He was in a state of quiet, almost passive enjoyment. All at once, without warning of any kind, he found himself wrapped around as it were by a flame-colored cloud. For an instant he thought of fire, some sudden conflagration in the great city, the next he knew that the light was within himself. Directly afterwards came upon him a sense of exultation, of immense joyousness accompanied or immediately followed by an intellectual illumination quite impossible to describe. Into his brain streamed one momentary lightning flash of the Brahmic Splendor which has ever since lightened his life; upon his heart fell one drop of Brahmic Bliss, leaving thenceforward for always an aftertaste of heaven. Among other things he did not come to believe, he saw and knew that the Cosmos is not dead matter but a living Presence, that the soul of man is immortal, that the universe is so built and ordered that without any peradventure all things work together for the good of each and all, that the foundation principle of the world is what we call love and that the happiness of every one is in the long run absolutely certain. He claims that he learned more within the few seconds during which the illumination lasted than in previous months or even years of study and that he learned much that no study could ever have taught.[61]

Though perhaps ultimately inexplicable, it seems clear that this experience was entirely consistent with Bucke's personality and with the transcendent optimism he had absorbed in varying degrees from theological and literary sources. More significantly, its influence was clearly evident in much of Bucke's published work on neuroscience.

Late in 1872, forced by ill health to discontinue his medical practice, Bucke searched for a less strenuous form of medical employment. It caused him little concern, for as he wrote to his friend Harry Forman, the government of Ontario planned to build an inebriate asylum and he expected to be appointed Medical Superintendent. "I consider I have almost a sure thing," he continued,

Mr. Pardee, who was with me in England last summer is now provincial secretary and the Asylums are all in his department. He is perhaps my most intimate friend here. He is very popular with the other members of the Government and in the House and he is to fix it.[62]

It was a reasonable expectation, for Bucke had spent many evenings playing poker with Pardee and was a vehement supporter of the party to which the Provincial Secretary belonged.[63]

Awaiting his appointment, Bucke earned a living speculating in oil, but all did not go well.[64] A year later he saw himself in "the position of a hanger-on waiting to have a bone thrown him" and could not see "that my individual prospects are at all advanced." The plan for the inebriate asylum was, in fact, indefinitely postponed, a decision that coincided with a fall in Canadian oil prices from three dollars a barrel to under seventy cents in 1873. Land prices fell accordingly and Bucke the speculator was forced to return, this time in partnership, to the practice of medicine.[65] After a year of practice he informed Forman that the institution for inebriates was to be opened, instead,

as a Lunatic Asylum, and I have a chance of the appointment if I want it, and I am not at all sure I shall want it. If other things go at all well with me I would not take it now.[66]

Whatever other interests Bucke hoped to take advantage of apparently did not materialize for, two months later, he sought testimonials from Sir William Jenner and Benjamin Ward Richardson in support of his application for the superintendency of the Hamilton Asylum. In February of 1876, he received his appointment and the following year transferred to London.[67]

It was the beginning of what was to be a quarter-century career in the asylum service, terminated only by accidental death in 1902.

He arrived as a political placeman, bringing no special training or, indeed, liking for psychiatric employment. His background was simply that of a well-trained general physician, an occupation that, in the 1870s, was schooled in the traditions of therapeutic skepticism and a clinical rather than experimental approach to medical learning. Yet the asylum was to provide Bucke with the opportunity to transcend these narrow medical confines, to expand them, in effect, so as to encompass current philosophical conceptions of the mind. Armed with this new synthesis of psychophysiological understanding, his years as a Medical Superintendent were marked by a variety of often controversial attempts to reconcile therapy with theoretical conviction.

2

The human ecology of the London Asylum

When Richard Maurice Bucke was appointed to the medical superintendency of the Hamilton Asylum in 1876 (Figure 6), he joined an institutional system rapidly emerging from a lengthy gestation. The first permanent asylum in Ontario had opened, with 500 patients, at Toronto in 1850 and, over the next dozen years, three branch asylums appeared in various makeshift premises. A vacant university building in Toronto received 61 patients in 1856, a converted barrack at Fort Malden on the Detroit River became home to 146 incurables in 1859, and 44 patients took up residence in a partially completed hotel at Orillia in 1861.[1] In that year, these institutions together housed 726 individuals, though additional patients were to be found in Kingston at the small Rockwood Asylum for the criminally insane. A decade later, however, after the transfer of patients from Malden and Orillia to the newly opened London Asylum, the number of patients under provincial care had nearly doubled. By 1881, with the conversion of Rockwood to a regular asylum and the opening of an institution in Hamilton, Ontario had charge of 2,652 persons of unsound mind.[2] The creation of three new institutions, together with accompanying legal procedures and inspection provisions, had, during the 1870s, transformed the province's resources for the insane from a single asylum to an extensive system of imposing institutions. By the end of the decade these asylums consumed 16.4% of the provincial budget, an amount that stablized at more than 19% in the late 1880s. Such a figure, in 1893, for example, was almost twice the combined provincial expenditure on penal institutions, general hospitals, houses of refuge, and orphanages.[3] The asylum, in effect, held pride of place in the provincial welfare system. It was both a symbol of state benevolence and official affirmation that to medicine had

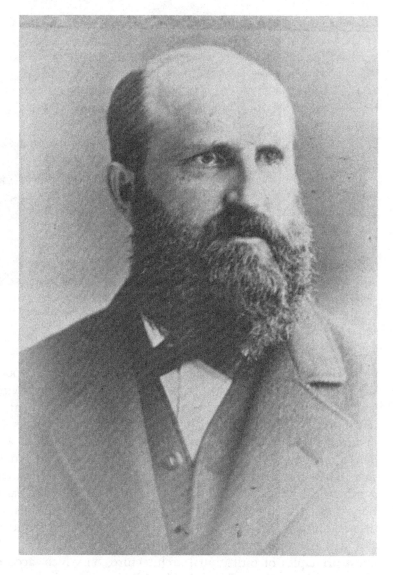

Figure 6. R. M. Bucke, c. 1876. Source: R. M. Bucke Collection, University of Western Ontario.

been delegated the task of defining the limits of normal thought and behavior.

The outward appearance of the London Asylum (Figure 7), to which Bucke was transferred after an unremarkable year in Ham-

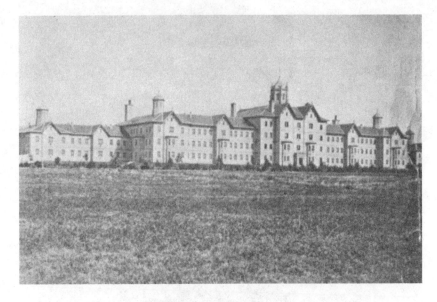

Figure 7. London Asylum, 1871. Source: London Psychiatric Hospital.

ilton, was calculated to stir a mixture of civic pride and therapeutic optimism in visiting citizenry. It was located on a 300-acre site, 3 miles east of the city, to which it was linked by telegraph and, after 1879, by "Professor Bell's new instrument, the telephone."[4] Surrounded by 50 acres of ornamental gardens, the institution was reached by a tree-lined avenue, 100 feet in width. The main building, of white brick and cut stone, capped by a slate roof, extended across a frontage of 610 feet from which symmetrical wings receded 220 feet to the rear. The central portion of the structure, four stories in height, housed administrative offices and quarters for medical staff and attendants. If the exterior was awesome in its size, the institution's interior adopted the latest principles of intitutional architecture, on which, according to the Inspector, "Asylums in the United States have recently been constructed." Steam heat, gas lighting, large wells producing one-half million gallons of water daily, 22-inch-diameter brick sewers, and strategic ventilator shafts combined to promise a maximum of sanitary comfort for the 900 patients lodged in the institution by 1878. Though linked to the main building by a covered passage, the Medical Superintendent's house (Figure 8),

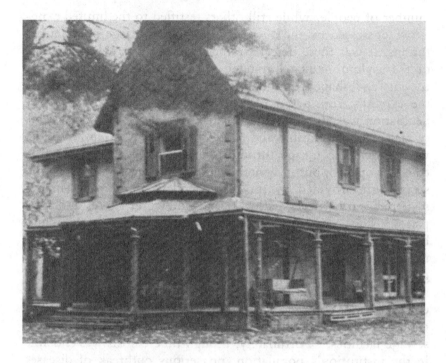

Figure 8. Medical Superintendent's house, London Asylum, n.d. (c. 1880). Source: London Psychiatric Hospital.

perhaps symbolically, stood apart, as did a large number of out-buildings associated with the 100-acre farm. A short distance to the north of the asylum proper stood three large brick cottages, each designed for 60 chronic patients, and a two-story structure housing 186 refractory patients.[5] Taken together, the various buildings of the London Asylum, as Bucke observed in 1883, "almost reached the magnitude of a town."[6] Indeed, the institution bore more than a physical resemblance to a village: It was, quite literally, a distinct community.

It was, however, a community the essence of which was not readily apparent to a casual observer. Despite both the grand exterior of the asylum, the largest building in the western half of the province, and the best intentions of the architect from the Public Works Department, the institution was plagued with or-ganizational and structural problems from its inception. Many of them were instrinsic to confined quarters housing a sizeable number of people, while still others testified to the limited experience possessed by the Victorian designers of large public institutions. It was these defects, rather than the external appearance of the asylum, which impinged most directly on the staff and patients and shaped the quality of their daily existence. Despite the carefully considered placement of windows, for example, ventilation was always deficient such that "bad air" and the odor of stale food permeated the halls.[7] In summer, offensive odors were allowed to escape through the few warped windows that could be opened, but in winter heat loss was the greater evil. The steam heat provided by four large boilers failed to warm the scattered wards, necessitating the use of wood stoves and fireplaces.[8] This procedure raised the temperature in the building, but brought with it, in Bucke's words, "great fear that should a fire ever get fairly started, the building would be burnt to the ground."[9] Indeed, in 1887, though no lives were lost, the extensive kitchen and laundry were entirely destroyed by fire.[10] An equally serious threat to the asylum inhabitants was the spread of contagious diseases by the omnipresent rats or by the inadequate sewage facilities.[11] Fortunately, though tuberculosis was endemic in the institution's population, no serious outbreak of diseases such as typhoid or cholera occurred during the late nineteenth century. Nonetheless, from the habitually leaking roof above to the worn softwood floor below,[12] the London Asylum, behind its imposing facade, offered a spartan standard of accommodation. Like the farms from which so many of the patients came, the institution found itself governed as much by weather conditions and the vegetative functions of aggregated humanity as by the intentions of its architects or physicians.

If the asylum's structure was not conducive to more than nominal comfort, its internal accoutrements did little to improve this standard. "As compared with most County Asylums in England," observed the visiting alienist, D. H. Tuke, "the furnishings of the main and north building struck me as somewhat scant." (Figure 9.) The "bare corridors and rooms" were considered adequate by the authorities, he continued, since "the patients of the class that go the London Asylum are not accustomed to more at home."[13] In the place of carpets or framed pictures, the patients were met by dim hallways and bare, though often crowded, wards. More significant were the barred windows,

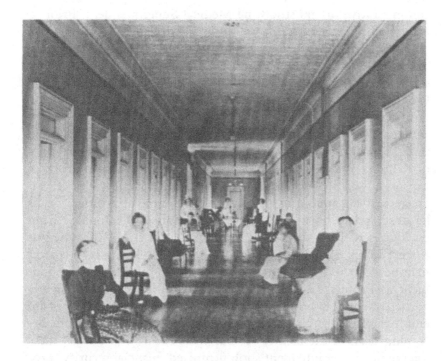

Figure 9. Female ward, London Asylum, 1911. Source: London Psychiatric Hospital.

locked wards, and exercise yards surrounded by a brick fence ten feet in height. Bucke was soon to discontinue the use of many of these restrictive appliances, but their continued presence served as a constant sign to the patients of their confined status within the asylum world.[14] It was an awareness that received frequent reemphasis from countless other aspects of the institution's furnishings. In 1882, for example, the Inspector authorized the replacement of the hard horsehair pillows for 100 of "the old and the sickly and feeble." It was trivial detail perhaps, but for the elderly patients uncomfortable bedding represented a nightly reminder of their institutionalization.[15] Indeed, the physical environment of the asylum, from its overbearing external dimensions to the individual patient's bed, reinforced in many subtle ways the anonymous dependency of the insane.

Far more complex than the institution's physical structure was the human ecology of the asylum. At the center of medical and administrative affairs stood the Medical Superintendent. Prior to his appointment, Bucke, it will be recalled, had viewed the office with some distaste.[16] He changed his mind rather quickly, however, in 1876, writing enthusiastically to Harry Forman, "my salary is $1,600.00 a year & House, Furniture, Fuel, Light & Provisions of all kinds found for myself & family so that the position is equal to about $4,000.00 a year."[17] Nor were the anticipated rewards of office entirely material. "It is a good thing," he wrote, "to have a situation where you have no superior officer within a hundred miles . . . I do my own work in my own way."[18] In addition to this independence, Bucke was aware that his appointment conferred a degree of prestige for, as he observed to Forman, "I have a position in the country from my duties which I would not have without them."[19] That he was correct in his estimation is suggested by his selection as a charter member of the Royal Society of Canada[20] and by his appointment as Professor of Nervous and Mental Disease at the newly created medical school in London.[21] Only the opposition of his employer, the provincial government, prevented him from becoming dean of the faculty several years later.[22] For Bucke, then, the medical superintendent's job promised financial security, professional independence, and prestige, both academic and social.

Initially, Bucke found his work "easy and pleasant" and noted that it "takes me on an average three or four hours a day."[23] Perhaps most uncongenial was the necessity of adapting to the rigid schedule which characterized asylum life. "I have to get up at six every morning," he complained to Harry Forman, "it is not really necessary except as an example – everybody in the house is supposed to be up at that hour and it would not do for me to stay in bed."[24] Gradually, his workload increased and a daily routine developed. Breakfast was followed by an hour or two in his office, after which, between 10:00 and 11:30, he made rounds of the wards with one of the assistant physicians. Afternoons were usually occupied by office work as were Saturday mornings.[25] The day concluded with early retirement for, as Bucke observed, his 6:00 rising "requires going to bed early thereby limiting social life."[26] Cloistered with his patients and subject to the same diurnal rhythm, Bucke quickly came to share what he referred to as "the horribly monotonous life of the patients."[27]

More subtle factors than early retirement, however, limited the

Medical Superintendent's social world. As will become apparent, his contact with the patients was usually hurried and impersonal, while his relation to the attendants was primarily in the guise of a disciplinarian. Only the bursar and the two or three assistant physicians provided relief from his isolation within the institution. Bucke was fortunate to develop a close friendship with the asylum bursar, a man whose eclectic interests mirrored his own. Charles Sippi was educated at Queen's College, Cork, and the Royal College of Surgeons, Dublin. He had practiced medicine for several years near London, taught classics, and managed a piano company before his asylum appointment. Music, in fact, was his principal interest and he was an able organist and choirmaster whose talents were often displayed at asylum entertainments.[28] Many evenings Bucke spent with Sippi and the assistant physicians discussing philosophy and playing whist. If Sippi found Bucke's departure from religious orthodoxy disconcerting, he enjoyed "his peculiar ways, his loud laugh, and his impulsiveness" and was clearly sensitive to his fluctuations in mood.[29] Since he reported directly to the Inspector, Sippi enjoyed a measure of equality with the Superintendent that may have paved the way for a friendship with which the other whist players would have been uncomfortable.

Over the years, in fact, Bucke's relationships with his assistant physicians appear to have been highly variable. Upon his appointment, for example, he was received with dislike by Dr. Stephen Lett, a favorite of the Inspector and heir-apparent upon the death of Bucke's predecessor. Apparently unaware of Lett's frustrated ambition, Bucke was distressed at the latter's rejection of his overtures. After he advised the Inspector that the hostile behavior of his subordinate jeopardized his own authority and that "all pretentions of friendship must cease," Lett was transferred to the Toronto Asylum.[30] Nor was this incident unique. Dr. Buchan and his family were accused of "unreasonable and vexatious expectations" of the asylum housemaids and of abuse of their food allocations. The family members, Bucke wrote, have "been for years the cause of ceaseless worries and troubles in whatever institutions they have been domiciled" and Buchan himself "is inert intellectually and takes no interest in the asylum service." The dispute simmered for three years, terminating in an investigation which could confirm none of the allegations and, instead, suggested Buchan was popular with most of the asylum attendants.[31] Less fortunate, however, was Dr. Burgess, who, it was said by two of his fellow assistant physicians, was the victim of a plot on the part of Bucke and a fourth assistant, Dr. Beemer. The Superintendent apparently complained of a "small rebellion" by Burgess, in order to allow Beemer to take the place of Burgess as senior assistant. Though the Inspector failed to document any rebellion, Burgess was transferred to the Hamilton Asylum and the other assistants were left in fear that a similar fate might eventually befall them.[32] Not all the assistant physicians were objects of the Superintendent's hostility. Dr. A. T. Hobbs, responsible for the asylum's gynecological surgery, won nothing but praise from Bucke.[33] In general, however, the assistants found themselves, like patients and attendants, dominated by the Superintendent and the daily constraints of institutional life. They lived at the asylum and were exposed to the same diet, diseases, and daily routine that governed the patients.[34] Salaries, even with board and lodging provided, were not competitive with private medical practice, and pensions not easily secured.[35] Permission to marry, because of the added institutional expense of maintaining dependents, could be arbitrarily denied by the Inspector,[36] while transfer to a distant institution could also be ordered at the Inspector's discretion.[37] Even more than was the case with Bucke, the assistant physicians were themselves creatures of an institution.

Eight years after his initial appointment, Bucke began to complain in his published reports of burdensome duties. The Medical Superintendent, he wrote,

is supposed to keep oversight of the buildings themselves as well as of the internal economy of *them,* the farm, garden grounds, repairs of all kinds, besides having care, medical and otherwise, of nine hundred patients; but no one man can keep in his mind and manage intelligently so many and such diverse details . . . .[38]

Though Inspector Langmuir had written that the agricultural and administrative affairs of the asylum were "second in importance to the care of the patients,"[39] the order of priority, if the allocation of the Superintendent's time is a guide, had clearly been reversed. His contact with patients was limited to rapid walking rounds of the wards, with detailed knowledge of cases left to the assistant physicians and attendants.[40] Instead, Bucke was inundated with administrative tasks, many of them painfully trivial.

In July of 1881, for example, a great deal of his time was spent investigating the alleged theft of a patient's parasol. Similarly, in 1895, correspondence rapidly accumulated with the Inspector, who had dismissed as "sensational" and "lascivious" novels by Conan Doyle or Wilkie Collins chosen by Bucke for the patients' library.[41] Record keeping was an equally tiresome but unavoidable task. All stores received by the asylum were eventually, after checking by the storekeeper and bursar, to be certified by the Superintendent.[42] Even more demanding was the compilation of statistical and descriptive material for the asylum's annual report. As Bucke wrote to Walt Whitman, "it seems the annual report fairly treads on the heels of the one in advance of it."[43] The burden of these administrative tasks was gradually to erode the professional identity that Bucke had brought to the asylum service. Indeed, as Inspector O'Reilly, himself a physician, remarked of the Superintendent, "his time is so fully occupied with outside matters (in which by education and training a medical man is not supposed to be most proficient) that he has very little time indeed to devote to those professional duties to which he is supposed to give the greater part of his attention."[44] The unfortunate metamorphosis of the North American physician turned asylum administrator, lamented by neurologists such as Edward Spitzka and Weir Mitchell, was to become a familiar criticism in medical circles during the final decades of the nineteenth century.[45] The critics, however, failed to recognize the dynamic significance of the process: Medical Superintendents, like their patients, were stripped of their pre-asylum identity and remodeled according to institutional imperatives.

By the 1890s, even the financial rewards of the superintendency began to pale. As Bucke wrote to his friend Horace Traubel, "the outlook is bad for anything more than a bare living. 5 boys and 2 girls to provide for is no joke."[46] Part of Bucke's difficulty arose from a poorly managed investment in his brother-in-law's water-meter company, an enterprise which, by 1892, was "absorbing money as a sandbank absorbs water" leaving him "a mere pauper."[47] By 1895, Bucke's salary was $2,000 and his various allowances for items such as rent, food, and domestic service added another $1,895.02, a total just under the $4,000 per annum of which he had boasted to Harry Forman two decades earlier.[48] It was a salary, as the Inspector noted, common to senior superintendents in Ontario, but representing only half that paid by the state of New York to its alienists.[49] Nor were the perquisites given overly generous. In 1892, the Inspector ordered that the diet of asylum officials was to be drawn from the stores used for the patients. Two years later, table supplies were formally restricted to a maximum of $50 a month and, subsequently, the allowance for household goods and furnishings restricted to $100 annually.[50] On matters ranging from requests for leave to suggestions for repairs to the Superintendent's house, the provincial authorities adopted increasingly inflexible procedures and regulations.[51]

Bucke had begun his career as a Medical Superintendent with little knowledge of insanity and had endorsed procedures he was later to disavow. He was, he recalled, "dogmatic in the inverse ratio of my experience."[52] Upon his appointment, he set about acquainting himself with the alienist's role, first, by touring American asylums in 1877, and secondly, by reading accepted authorities on mental pathology, such as Henry Maudsley and Daniel H. Tuke.[53] Whatever his hopes of shaping the asylum and its inmates, however, in the long run the relationship was to prove at least reciprocal. As adminstrative tasks accumulated, he was gradually stripped of all but the outward remnants of his medical identity. Forced to share food and living space with his charges, their daily routine quickly became his. Isolated from the medical and social life of nearby London, his friendships and animosities were restricted to a small circle of asylum officials. Like his patients and attendants, Bucke's existence was governed by the will of the Inspector and the regulations formulated by the provincial government. And finally, with no alternative livelihood, such as a carefully nurtured medical practice readily at hand, Bucke had only the prospect of continued asylum service so as to secure a modest pension on retirement.[54] Nominally the controlling voice of the asylum, the Medical Superintendent was as much governed as governor.

In formal terms, the Medical Superintendent was directly responsible to the Inspector of Prisons and Public Charities. This official mediated, on the one hand, between Bucke and the provincial government, in the person of the Provincial Secretary, and on the other, between Bucke and his staff and patients. The former role was primarily legislative, that is, informing the government of necessary statutes to be passed in the legislature, advising on orders-in-council, or formulating regulations autonomously under existing legislation. The latter role was acquitted largely during the three annual visits to the asylum, at which time the premises were inspected, accounts reviewed, the patients seen by roll call, and complaints from attendants investigated.[55] With the exception of his close friendship with Thomas Pardee, to whom he owed his initial appointment, Bucke had little direct contact with the Provincial Secretary, the minister in charge of the asylum system. His relationship with the inspectors appointed during his tenure was much more direct, and varied significantly in tone. During the 1880s, W. T. O'Reilly, formerly Provincial Inspector for Insurance, was a warm supporter of Bucke and his innovations at London.[56] He was succeeded in 1890, by Robert Christie, who brought to his inspections a far more critical and sometimes hostile perspective.[57] Undoubtedly the most dynamic Inspector, however, was J. W. Langmuir, the first official appointed under the Prison and Asylum Inspection Act by the newly created province of Ontario in 1868. Arriving from Scotland at age fifteen, he quickly became a successful merchant and municipal politician in eastern Ontario. When only thirty-three, he was appointed to the inspectorship and for the next fourteen years the asylums fell under his energetic scrutiny. In 1882 he resigned to become manager of the Toronto General Trust Company, an organization that supervised the estates of many of Ontario's asylum patients, and later became president of the Homewood Retreat Association, which owned a private asylum in Guelph.[58] It was during Langmuir's tenure that the daily affairs of the emerging Ontario asylum system took shape.

The periodic instrusions of the Inspector into Bucke's London empire were often disquieting experiences for the Superintendent. On occasion these visits took the form of outright confrontations,[59] but more often they simply resulted in, as Bucke observed, "a devil of a stack of work."[60] During some inspections, though by no means all, the Inspector "went over the patients' muster roll, and saw, and conversed with each one separately."[61] It was "quite a chore," Bucke observed, "to call the roll of over 900 people,"[62] many of whom were doubtless scarcely known to him. More frequently, the Inspector concentrated his attention on patients who bore the marks of physical violence in order to rule out the possibility of mistreatment.[63] Attendants as well as patients were interviewed and disputes adjudicated.[64] Most visits resulted in demands for more exact record keeping, on matters as diverse as the use of patient restraints or the receipt of supplies, and in orders to improve standards of maintenance or cleanliness in various areas of the asylum.[65] Bucke's asylum was, it is clear, by no means as free from outside interference as he had led Harry Forman to believe.

Beneath the Inspector's seemingly picayune criticisms lay a much deeper concern. To be sure, he was sensitive to the welfare of asylum patients and was rigorous in investigating any hint of mistreatment. But more important still was a preoccupation with the relentless growth of the asylum system and with the costs of its maintenance. It was a concern that doubtless reflected accurately the priorities of a government faced with a slow but inexorable increase in the proportion of provincial funds devoted to asylums. Unlike Britain and some American states, provision for the insane had been recognized from the beginning as a provincial rather than local expense. By the late 1870s it was, as the Inspector observed:

quite evident that more careful discrimination will have to be exercised in granting admission or the vacant beds will very soon be filled with chronic and incurable subjects, many of whom are sent to the Asylum, not because they are dangerous or even troublesome, but simply because their relatives want to get rid of them.[66]

Patients were received through the courts on a warrant, signifying a potentially dangerous individual and requiring immediate incarceration, or by a certificate, bearing the signature of two physicians and simply indicating a person of unsound mind.[67] The latter class were, the Inspector felt, often "harmless and incurable and . . . therefore could be taken care of in the family." As a result, the medical superintendent was given limited discretionary power to refuse admission to these individuals unless they had a remedial condition, were a threat to life or property, or had no family able to care for them.[68] Such selectivity, however, was potentially circumvented by determined relatives who could gain mandatory admission by avoiding certificates and, through testimony as to the obstreperous character of the patient, securing a warrant instead.[69] Despite the desire to limit

Table 2.1. *Asylum populations in Ontario and at London, selected years*

Year	Total daily average asylum pop. in Ont.	Ont. pop.	Patient rate per 1,000 pop.	London Asylum pop.	London as % of Ont. total
1871	1366	1,620,851	0.84	457	33
1881	2584	1,926,922	1.34	852	33
1891	3888	2,114,321	1.84	974	25
1901	5256	2,182,947	2.41	1034	20

Sources: M.C. Urquhart and K.C. Buckley, *Historical Statistics of Canada* (Cambridge: 1965) 14; IR, 1903, IX; 1892, 6; 1902, XIV; ARMS, 1882, 75; 1872, 165)

admissions at the London Asylum, the Inspector stated in 1885, "904 beds are always kept filled, and there are always applications for admission awaiting vacancies as they occur from discharges and death."[70] Indeed, the number of patients in the Ontario system increased from 1 per 1,187 residents in 1871 to 1 in 547 by 1891[71] (Table 2.1).

If the Inspector was unable to curtail the asylum's growth, his alternative goal became the economical administration of each institution. "It is important," he warned Bucke, "that the exact cost, under every heading of maintaining lunatics in each Department of this Asylum should be known."[72] Costs were, indeed, monitored diligently but the yearly amount required to support the London institution increased from 3.15% of the provincial budget in 1878 to 3.6% in 1893[73] (Tables 2.2 and 2.3). Generally less than 1% of the cost per patient represented expenditures on medicines and "medical comforts,"[74] which suggested that economies could be achieved through measures such as increased farm productivity or by encouraging relatives to clothe the patients.[75] A potentially promising tactic was to secure payment from those patients with known resources. It was the bursar's duty to inquire into the ability of a patient or the patient's family to contribute at least a portion of the weekly upkeep.[76] The proportion of paying patients never exceeded 12–15% of the total at London and the average amount paid by each was little

Table 2.2. *Expenditures, London and Ontario Aslyums, 1868–93*

Year	All asylums as % total Ont. welfare expenditure	London Asylum as % total welfare expenditure	All asylums as % total provincial expenditure	London Asylum as % total prov. expend.
1868	62.4	–	15.0	–
1878	55.6	10.6	16.4	3.1
1888	60.2	10.9	19.2	3.5
1893	58.7	11.2	19.0	3.6

Source: R. Splane, *Social Welfare in Ontario, 1791–1893* (Toronto: 1965), 282–3; IR, 1878, 24; 1888, 19; 1893, 18.

Table 2.3 *Asylum expenditures and total provincial expenditures, selected years*

Year	Provinicial expenditure	All asylum expenditure	Expenditures per patient	London Asylum expenditures	Expenditure per patient
1878	2,784,321	270,162.95	125.72	87,394.84	134.14
1888	3,536,248	459,373.39	144.38	122,692.56	134.53
1893	3,907,145	568,495.25	154.73	141,546.63	144.34

Source: R. Splane, *Social Welfare in Ontario, 1791–1893* (Toronto: 1965), 283; IR, 1878, 24; 1888, 32–3; 1893, 18, 4.

more than two-thirds the cost of their annual maintenance. In fact, despite formal agreements as to weekly payments, a significant proportion of the patients quickly defaulted and the list of arrears grew accordingly.[77] Though commodity prices fell gradually over the last quarter of the century and wages remained generally stable,[78] the Inspector's best efforts could not prevent a persistent annual increase in the cost of maintaining Ontario asylums. Indeed, by the end of the 1880s, they consumed almost one-fifth of the provincial budget.[79]

While the provincial government may well have found the increased costs of asylums distressing, such facilities, legislators knew, performed a useful role as welfare institutions. Not only was this seen as of practical benefit to the indigent, but it also symbolized the largesse of a benevolent government. Beyond such concerns, however, the asylums served a more covert but significant role for politicians: They were an important source of patronage. Bribery in order to secure supply contracts was not unknown[80] and local merchants of the correct political affiliation expected asylum accounts as a matter of course. Wrote one rebuffed businessman to the Inspector: "It seems that a life-long political allegiance and servitude counts for nothing, in my particular case, with your department; for favours are shown and advantages given to parties who never have once voted for the present Ontario Government."[81] That this angry individual had been overlooked may have been an exception, at least in the view of the antigovernment London *Free Press*, which complained that bids were seldom sought but rather, money was spent at "the wise discretion of Dr. Bucke" and "the Liberal Junta at Toronto."[82] Perhaps even more common than the partisan allocation of supply tenders was the placement of political supporters in the asylum service. "These political appointments are a nuisance," complained the bursar, "the efficiency of the institution is a secondary consideration." He looked forward to a day "when men will be appointed on their merits, not on their politics."[83] Occasionally the appointment of "highly recommended" persons was done on a direct ministerial request.[84] More often, local politicians sought favors at the asylum. T. S. Hobbs, for example, a successful merchant and the Liberal member of the legislature for London, wrote to advise the reinstatement of a dismissed attendant. "His relatives here are good supporters of mine," he explained, "and I am anxious to conciliate them by doing everything in my power for their brother."[85] That his appeal succeeded,[86] though the employee in question had been discharged for striking a patient, is indicative of the extent to which the operation of the London Asylum was subject to direct political interference. In this sense, it served a widely known and accepted social role.

The London Asylum, then, was officially dominated by a hierarchy beginning with the Provincial Secretary and passing via the Inspector, to the Superintendent, the bursar, and the assistant physicians. The members of this group, in fact, were molded to a single purpose. The Superintendent and, to a lesser extent, his junior colleagues found the significant aspects of their medical role all but absent. The diagnosis of insanity was already made when the patient arrived at the institution, leaving only the often arbitrary task of classification. While under asylum care, as the accumulation of chronic cases suggested, few patients were treated with effective result. Stripped of the diagnostic and therapeutic function, the alienist found his opportunities for professional recognition beyond the asylum service closely circumscribed.[87] "Your hospitals are not our hospitals," Dr. Weir Mitchell told North American asylum superintendents, "Your ways are not our ways."[88] Instead, the superintendent's role had become bureaucratized, had, in effect, espoused the ethos of the inspector. His perspective centered on the institution itself rather than on the individuals who inhabited it. As the state's watchdog, he was dedicated to cost-efficient management, to the provision of a minimum standard of care for the indigent at a minimum level of expenditure by the more affluent. In pursuit of this objective, the asylum population was rationalized, with separate institutions created for such distinct dependent categories as the blind or the mentally deficient. Within the asylum, the inspector insisted that standardized, centralized regulations replace ad hoc, decentralized, decision making and that meticulous records, especially financial, be kept of all institutional affairs. The specialization of employee function was encouraged, as was the absolute control over employees exercised by the Superintendent through manipulation of wages or the power of rapid dismissal.[89] And though patronage considerations certainly intruded on the affairs of the asylum, the system was, in the interest of efficiency, nonpartisan to the extent that no political party contemplated its radical alteration or demise.[90] These management precepts were to blossom, in North America, with evangelic enthusiasm in the rhetoric of Frederick W. Taylor and his Progressive era followers.[91] But the roots of this credo, this blend of efficiency and uplift, may be traced into the 1870s as governments coped with the bureaucratic implications of what had once seemed brave social experiments.[92] As for asylums, the often tenuous distinction between medicine and social policy had been formally obliterated with the bureaucratization of the institutional physicians.

As the medical hierarchy became inextricably linked with administrative functions, its isolation from patients increased. Indeed, in terms of affluence, education, and power physicians had always been alienated from their often indigent charges in the public asylums. To fill the vacuum that characterized the institutional doctor–patient relationship, the daily contact with patients devolved upon the asylum's attendants.[93] From the early nineteenth century there had, of course, been an important role assigned to the nonmedical staff. According to the theory of therapy that became known as moral treatment,[94] constant personal contact with the patients by empathetic keepers was the key to recovery. Attendants would, in effect, by the very force of their reasoned personalities, urge their charges back to sanity. Ignoring the potential threat to medical supremacy that was implicit in the essential role accorded laymen,[95] English alienists such as John Conolly at the Hanwell Asylum argued that successful implementation of a nonrestraint system required no less than one attendant for every fifteen patients.[96] As asylums grew in size, the role of the keeper increased in significance, not as an agent of moral treatment, but rather, as a simple custodian. Beyond this formal function, moreover, in their daily interaction with patients, as in general hospitals, "attendants helped shape a hospital subculture" quite distinct from that familiar to the medical hierarchy.[97] Since little documentation remains as to the nature of this subculture, its character must be inferred "from chance remarks and patterns of institutional practice."[98] Attendants, then, were central to both the recognized institutional routines and the covert infrastructure of nineteenth-century asylums.[99]

In the London Asylum, the ratio of attendants to patients, by the late 1880s, was one to thirteen, a proportion quite acceptable by Conolly's standard.[100] Less appropriate, apparently, was the character of these attendants. "At present the employment is taken up casually and temporarily," complained Bucke in 1886, "just as the person might take service on a farm or in a shop." Drawn from the same social circumstances as the patients, the attendants may have been able to slip into easy relationships with their charges. But Bucke was oblivious to this quality and argued, to the contrary, that the keepers lacked any "special fitness for the work." In order to "elevate the standard and increase the efficiency" of attendants, he suggested screening prospective employees for temperament, intelligence, and education, and initiating for those who met the mark "special teaching in the form of lectures and examinations" by the asylum physicians.[101] It was an approach calculated to replace the commonsense view of insanity, which informed the attendant subculture, with a distinctly medical perspective. Such schemes, indeed, were frequently proposed by Anglo-American alienists. Many English medical superintendents gave private lectures to their staff, a process that Bucke began in 1891.[102] The Medico–Psychological Association in Britain supplemented such ad hoc training by the publication of the *Handbook for Attendants of the Insane* in 1885 (a text that the London asylum eventually acquired in 1902), and by a formal certification examination after 1891.[103] In the United States, training for nurses intending to work with the mentally ill began in 1882 at the McLean Hospital in Boston, and twelve such facilities appeared in New York state alone by the end of the century.[104] But this professionalization process scarcely influenced Canadian asylums in the nineteenth century. Indeed, the most sophisticated preparation Bucke sought in prospective attendants was a knowledge of music so as to ensure participation in asylum entertainments.[105]

The duties that these untrained individuals were expected to perform were, in theory, relatively uncomplicated. An attendant was assigned to a specific ward housing patients of the same sex, a brief experiment using woman keepers on a male ward having failed.[106] Each activity of the day that required patients to leave the ward, including mealtimes, work parties, and evening entertainment, demanded close supervision by the attendants stationed in various strategic areas. They were expected to prevent both violence between patients and any ill-advised attempts at escape.[107] Their authority was enhanced and their social kinship with the patients presumably diminished with the introduction of uniforms in 1881.[108] While on the wards, the attendants assisted patients in matters of hygiene, reported on behavior and accidents to the medical staff, and provided such nursing care as was required by the aged or infirm. On two evenings a week during the fall and winter, employees were required to attend dances and were explicitly instructed to dance with patients.[109] On other evenings they were obliged to be present at entertainment staged in the dining hall, and on Sunday were expected to participate in church service.[110] Many employees lived at the asylum and whether they actually took their meals with the patients or in a separate attendants' dining room, the standard of fare differed little from that of the patients.[111] The attendants were, in fact, plagued by a fundamental ambiguity. On the one hand, they shared with the patients both a common social origin and an identical daily routine, while on the other, as uniformed disciplinarians, they were charged with the detailed supervision of the patients' lives.[112]

The tension inherent in the attendants' role did not go unremarked. "You are closely confined," Bucke himself admitted, "your hours of duty are very long, and your patience and temper are often severely tried."[113] Recalling with appreciation social contacts between staff and patients, a former patient sympathized with the attendants' plight. "How lonely the attendants must be sometime," he wrote, "shut up for days and weeks, and even years with only a few hours freedom."[114] Perhaps the most eloquent statement of the frustration associated with the attendants' post came in 1879 from Mr. Meek, the Chief Attendant and senior employee:

Our position . . . is a very peculiar one, and can only be thoroughly appreciated by those conversant with the nature of the hell demon of insanity. A daily residence of fifteen hours in the midst of beings from whom all that is human and good seems to be separated, leaving behind only the semblance of God's image, with the nature of Frankenstein, has a very dark side. There is a constant struggle to remember that it is the disease and not the mind that speaks and acts, combined with a never ending effort to maintain a cheerful and kind demeanor towards those for whose bodily care we are responsible. . . . A momentary lapse, a seemingly slight oversight almost surely entails dismissal, most certainly a severe reprimand, which to the unfortunate attendant striving to do his duty is doubly severe.[115]

The medical staff and many patients would doubtless have conceded the accuracy of Meek's anguished description. Attendants were constantly caught between the demands of their position and the reality of life in the patient subculture. Many, as will be seen, either became casualties or, more often, chose to abandon the struggle.[116]

Neither wages nor conditions of employment were calculated to recompense attendants adequately for the uncongenial nature of their post.[117] Though provision was made for paid sick leave for long-term employees, other perquisites were less attractive. When attendants complained of the standard of board, improvements were instituted, but the repetitive menu remained that of a parsimonious institution.[118] In 1887 the government abruptly decided that the provision of accommodation for the families of married attendants imposed a "large and cumbersome" burden. Denying an intent "to take hasty action . . . or to deal harshly with those concerned," the Inspector ordered all families to leave the institution within six months. No married staff were to be hired in future and "in the course of time" the services of those already married would "be dispensed with."[119] Even for single employees, however, employment was uncongenial, due largely to low wages. In 1882, Bucke complained that wage rates had generally risen in the province, leaving the asylum scale unattractive. A female attendant, for example, was paid ten dollars monthly and was given board; in private domestic service, she might earn a somewhat lower wage but would work far fewer hours and enjoy a significantly more attractive standard of living.[120] Bucke's concern for wage rates was clearly less directed to the welfare of his staff than to the difficulty in securing sufficient employees to meet institutional needs.[121] When the economy entered a recession in the 1890s, asylum wages appeared relatively more attractive. Male attendants earned twenty dollars a month, in addition to board, a figure substantially better than that paid to farm or general laborers and approximately equivalent to that commanded in such skilled trades as carpentry.[122] "Judging by the great number of applications," wrote Bucke, "I feel no doubt we could get as good attendants as at present for the smaller salary." Indeed, he continued, a lower salary would still attract young men but, after a brief time, compel them to leave, thereby preventing the accumulation of "middle aged and elderly men" on the asylum staff.[123] Despite the significant role played by the attendants in ongoing patient care, their status in the eyes of the asylum hierarchy, reflected in their remuneration, was never more than marginal.

The result of low wages and uncongenial working conditions was to produce a significant resignation rate in the London Asylum. Between 1876 and 1881, an average of 21 employees, out of a total of approximately 102, resigned each year.[124] Similarly, of the 31 attendants engaged between 1892 and 1894, 18 remained in 1895 with the average length of service of the group amounting to a scant 14.5 months[125] (Table 2.4). Many perhaps saw no possibility of betterment, for promotion brought a relatively small increase in salary, few perquisites, and often entailed un-

Table 2.4. *Turnover in London Asylum attendants, 1877–97*

Year	Total attendants	Reason for leaving			Length of service[a] (years)					
		Discharged	Resigned	Transferred or died	<1	1–2	2–4	4–6	6–8	8>
1877	(1878–83)	17	20	2	23	4	8	4	0	4
1887	70	13	13	1	17	1	6	0	0	2
1897	87	3	11	0	6	4	4	0	0	0

[a]The discrepancies between these figures and the total number of employees leaving the asylum appears in the original records.
Source: Ontario Archives, Rg.10, 20-C-4, Vol. 1, London Asylum, Register of Employees, 1870–1923; IR, 1878, 61; 1887, 21; 1897, 23.

pleasant responsibilities. Moreover, since supervisory jobs were awarded on the basis of seniority, with only special difficulties such as illiteracy barring their receipt, they carried little in the way of prestige.[126] Lacking such financial and status incentives, the attendant positions appeared to attract predominantly the transient and unskilled. They brought with them few of the special qualities sought by the Medical Superintendent and, instead, often seemed inept or insensitive. In fact, as the attendants watched over the patients the medical staff found it necessary to scrutinize the attendants. "Eyes and ears must be everywhere," wrote Bucke's predecessor, Dr. Henry Landor, "to prevent some kind of abuse or other among seventy servants."[127]

Upon his arrival at the London Asylum in 1877, Bucke's behavior suggested he had little need of Landor's warning. "During the first two or three months of my residence," he wrote, "I discharged a good many attendants."[128] Seventeen of the employees were dismissed[129] for failing to meet the conditions of tenure which Bucke outlined at the annual ball. The qualities he demanded included sobriety, obedience, honesty, morality, diligence, regular attendance, and a nonviolent attitude toward patients.[130] Such tractable saints were, in reality, seldom forthcoming, and a significant proportion of Bucke's administrative duties involved disciplining attendants. Dereliction of duty during night watch was a common cause of dismissal.[131] More serious, but not uncommon, was violence toward patients, whether in the subtle guise of the unwarranted use of restraint, or in the form of direct abuse. Those cases that could be documented resulted in routine dismissal and occasional criminal proceedings.[132] Similarly, cases of theft usually involved formal charges, and, in one instance, plunged Bucke into libel litigation.[133] Periodically, accusations of sexual impropriety were documented, either between attendants, or between attendants and patients, in all cases resulting in dismissal.[134] Finally, drunkenness was an offense sufficiently common among both attendants and support staff that discharge was not invariably the result.[135] In general, it appears that the most common cause of dismissal was neglect of or absence from duty, followed in order by mistreatment of patients, immoral conduct, and drunkenness.[136]

How, then, did attendants fit into the human geography of the asylum? As one patient astutely observed, it was often "difficult to distinguish the sane from the insane, the officer from the patient."[137] This perception testified to the common social origins of patients and attendants and to their shared institutional routine. From Bucke's perspective, attendants represented not his noble ideal but rather "the lowest class of labour."[138] Attempts were made, using educational tactics and uniforms, to differentiate between patients and staff but, because of the high turnover rate, to little avail. Despite the failure to drive a permanent medical wedge between keepers and kept, "it must be born in mind," the Inspector warned, "that while medical officers enter the Asylum wards from once to twice daily, attendants have the patients continually under supervision," and are responsible for administering whatever personal treatments the physicians ordered.[139] It was from this contact that a subculture emerged, a relationship doubtless woven of rules broken, punishments dispensed, food denied or allocated, or liberties permitted. It was a system of interactions in many ways as closed to the superintendent's scrutiny as it is to that of historians. And finally, the attendants, themselves, though little remains of their making, were hardly mute and passive. Many expressed themselves by resignation or through actions known to provoke dismissal. Still others used the asylum to their own advantage. They sought brief employment at the institution as a strategy by which to withstand a period of economic adversity or to secure a steppingstone to a more lucrative post. Some were more articulate. The asylum farmer, Bucke recalled with a note of incredulity, "informed me that it was a common impression that if 'I was locked up for a few months myself it would do me good.' "[140] The distinctions, it seems, between attendants, patients, and physicians were often indistinct and, as in a madhouse, occasionally turned upside down.

The frequently divergent perspectives of attendants and the medico-administrative hierarchy converged, ultimately, upon the patients. When Bucke assumed the superintendency in 1877, 623 inmates resided at the London Asylum, a population exceeded by only a dozen of the largest institutions on the continent. During the 1890s from 100 to 200 cases were admitted yearly and the total number of patients grew to over 1,000.[141] Who were the people who comprised this legion of lunatics, the individuals for whom the asylum became a home, a place to die, or a refuge

from a heartless world? While it is inaccurate "to translate archival silence into historical passivity,"[142] the reconstruction of the
patients' indentities, let alone their perceptions, is far more difficult than in the case of attendants. Indeed, that so little descriptive material remains is in itself suggestive of the inmates' anonymous status within the asylum. Only after Bucke's arrival were
regular casebooks kept in which the details of each admission
were entered and added to during the patient's hospitalization.[143]
Typical entries recorded relatively sterile data such as age, marital
status, nationality, and religion. In some cases brief note was
made of precipitating causes, the presence of hereditary factors,
whether the patient was admitted by certificate or warrant, and
the amount, if any, to be paid for upkeep. In few cases were
detailed descriptions given of appearance, behavior, previous illness, or the events preceding admission. Scant though this ad-
mitting information was, it was far more than was usually recorded later in the patient's career. Subsequent entries either
documented accidents, physical illnesses, and misbehavior or,
more commonly, were dated January 1st of each year and simply
read: "Remains unchanged bodily & mentally since this time last
year."[144] Beside one such 1894 notation, in fact, an exasperated
assistant physician had scribbled: "This patient is recorded as
having died 8 August, 1892. Under these circumstances I am not
sufficiently 'up' in the mysteries of spiritualism to 'call her back'
and continue the history."[145] This sardonic marginalia captured
the quintessential faceless patient. While a proportion of the acute
cases recovered and quickly departed, a great many patients sank
into chronic anonymity, leaving behind only occasional traces on
patterns of institutional practice.

Patients arrived at the London Asylum by one of two routes.
In 58% of the admissions to Ontario institutions between 1876
and 1896, patients were received on a medical certificate. This
document, often originating in the family, required the signature
of two physicians and eventuated in admission at the discretion
of the Superintendent according to available space. The remaining portion of patients were given mandatory admission on the
basis of a Lieutenant-Governor's warrant signifying an individual
dangerous to self or others. To obtain this document, relatives,
friends, or civil authorities placed information before a Justice of
the Peace who, if satisfied, committed the person to jail. There,

the jail surgeon and one other physician, if in agreement, issued a certificate and the county judge was required to do likewise. These certificates were reviewed for completeness by the Department of the Provincial Secretary, which then requested the Inspector to issue a warrant for the transfer of the patient from the jail to an asylum. In 1892, an average of eighteen days elapsed between the initial incarceration and transfer to an asylum, while in 1896, of the 1,888 persons committed to jail, 323 recovered there or were declared not to be insane.[146]

Despite the large volume of paper work associated with asylum committal, however, the documents were seldom informative. According to Inspector W.T. O'Reilly:

The cause as stated in each case is gathered from the so-called history of the case, which accompanies the medical certificate on the admission of each patient. The statement made as to 'causes' in these cases are, very often, of small value for various reasons – such as the want of knowledge of facts, carelessness in stating them, or a desire on the part of relatives to conceal important facts which should be told. Again, if a patient has been addicted to any particular vice or excess, or had recently suffered from any important accident or illness, one of these, right or wrong is set down as the cause of the insanity; and as these histories were generally written by unskilled persons, it will be easily understood that they are, when so written, of little value.[147]

Indeed, asylum officials were unable in 1879, to identify a predisposing cause for insanity in 71% of cases or an exciting cause in 43%, figures which remained unchanged over the next decade[148] (Table 2.5). Such vague information as to the reason for committal makes an assessment of the patient's admission status difficult. It does suggest, however, as Inspector O'Reilly commented, that the reason for admission was often not grossly abnormal or violent behavior but, rather, a desire on the part of the patient's "friends . . . to free themselves of the care and expense of their demented and comparatively harmless relatives." The disproportionate prominence of the elderly in the asylum population furnishes an example of the Inspector's concern.[149] From 1891 to 1895, 11.6% of admissions to Ontario asylums were over 65 years old, an age group representing only 4.6% of the general population. Such patients were often suffering from "senile decay," a term signifying not threatening behavior but confusion and forgetfulness of varying severity. For them the

Table 2.5. *Assigned causes of insanity on admission,*
selected years

Cause	1880 Predisposing/ exciting	1890 Predisposing/ exciting	1900 Predisposing/ exciting/ both
Moral	2/57	0/33	1/26/15
Physical	10/50	2/53	21/37/33
Hereditary	40/ –	30/ –	55/ –/ 5
Congenital	0/ –	0/ –	1/ –/ 0
Unknown	108/53	113/60	25/40/ 0
Total admissions	160	145	156

Source: ARMS, 1880, 325; 1890, 86; 1900, 55.

Table 2.6. *Duration of patient incarceration, selected years*

Years	1880 N	%	1890 N	%	1900 N	%
0–1	117	15	126	13	106	11
1–2	86	11	48	5	68	7
2–4	119	15	91	10	114	11
4–10	228	29	251	27	278	28
10+	234	30	430	46	442	44

Source: IR, 1880, 55; 1890, 13; 1900, xxiii.

prospect of recovery was slim and they remained as permanent inhabitants while younger patients were discharged. By the mid-1890s, chronic cases had accumulated to the point where, in the Inspector's view, they accounted for 90% of the asylum's inhabitants. In fact, in 1890, almost three-quarters of the patients had been resident for over four years, and almost one-half more than ten years[150] (Table 2.6). It appears, then, that a major reason for admission was the inability or unwillingness of friends, family, or community to cope in alternative fashion with harmless but chronically disorderly and unproductive behavior.[151]

How may the average patient be characterized? (Table 2.7.)

Table 2.7. *Patient characteristics, compared by percentage[a] to Ontario population, selected years*

Characteristic	1880–1 Asylum	Ont.	1890–1 Asylum	Ont.	1900–1 Asylum	Ont.
1. Sex						
a. male	49	51	49	51	49	50
b. female	51	49	51	49	51	50
2. Marital						
a. married	44	32	56	33	54	35
b. single	43	64	43	62	46	60
c. widowed	12	4	1	4	0	5
3. Religion						
a. Protestant	79	67	74	71	77	69
b. Roman Catholic	12	17	14	17	14	18
c. Other, unknown	14	16	11	13	9	13
4. Birthplace						
a. Canada	48	78	18	81	83	86
b. Ireland	15	7	11	5	3	3
c. England/Scotland	26	11	68	10	13	9
d. U.S.A.	4	2	1	2	2	1
e. Other	7	2	2	2	0	1
5. Occupation[b]						
i. male						
a. farmer	37	23	44	31	40	15
b. laborer	29	8	18	4	22	39
c. professional	3	?	1	?	1	5
d. other	22	?	31	?	40	?
e. none, unknown, huckster	7	?	3	?	3	?
ii. female						
a. servant	11	2	14	3	13	48
b. domestic duties	63	?	76	?	62	
c. professional	0	?	0	?	3	?
d. other	7	?	4	?	20	?
e. unknown, none, prostitute	16	?	7	?	3	?

[a]to nearest percentage.
[b]Male calculated as percentage of male patients and general population, similarly for female patients. Census data for occupations of women is incomplete; 1900–1 Ontario figures calculated as percentage of wage earners by sex.
Sources: ARMS, 1880, 317, 323–4; 1890, 78, 83–5; 1900, 48, 53–4; Canada Census, 1800–1, vol. 1, 97, 203, 398–9; vol. 2, 280–315; 1890–1, vol. 1, 144, 252–3, 363; vol. 2, 163–9; 1900–1, vol. 1, 52–3, 184, 416–7, Census (1901) Bulletin No. 1,1907, 3–4.

Table 2.8. *Age of patients admitted to London Asylum, compared to distribution of ages in Ontario by percentage, selected years*[a]

| | 1890–1 | | 1900–1 | |
Age	Asylum	Census	Asylum	Census
up to 20	14	46	4	42
20 to 40	49	32	53	32
40 to 60	30	17	31	18
over 60	7	7	12	7
unknown	0	0	1	0

[a]to nearest percentage.
Sources: IR, 1890, 27; 1900, *xxxix*; Canada Census, 1890–1, vol. 2, 6–9; 1900–1, vol. 2, 8–11.

Approximately equal numbers of male and female patients were admitted, a reflection not of the incidence of mental illness, but of the segregated accommodation provided at the asylum. Slightly more patients were married than single, while in the Ontario population in general (largely due to the many persons under twenty), the number of single individuals significantly exceeded those who were married. As the century drew to a close, the proportion of patients born in Canada, as would be expected, increased. Of the foreign born, the English and Scottish always accounted for the largest proportion, followed by persons born in Ireland, in a pattern similar to the composition of the Ontario population as a whole. Roman Catholics generally comprised less than 15% of the admissions, with Methodists and Presbyterians, as in the general population, slightly more prominent than the Church of England patients, among the Protestants. Relatively few patients under twenty years of age or over sixty were admitted to the asylum, the greatest number of cases falling in the twenty-to-forty age group. Approximately a quarter of the patients were admitted from Middlesex County (Table 2.8) in which the asylum was located, with another 50% originating in contiguous or nearby counties. Finally, from 1870 to 1900, among male patients, by far the most common occupations were farmer (41%) or laborer (25%), while female patients were frequently housewives (57%) or domestics (14%)[152] (Table 2.9).

Table 2.9. *County of residence, London Asylum admissions, selected years*

County of residence	Number of patients admitted		
	1880	1890	1900
Middlesex	40	39	43
Huron	18	12	19
Lambton	12	17	12
Essex	11	10	9
Elgin	10	8	12
Oxford	18	15	8
Perth	14	10	20
Kent	17	16	18
Total yearly admissions	140	145	156
Eight counties as percentage of total admissions	87.5	87.5	90.3

Source: ARMS, 1880, 318; 1890, 79; 1900, 49.

While more detailed statistical study might reveal otherwise hidden correlations between the preceding characteristics,[153] the most significant quality – poverty – is undoubtedly best documented from manuscript sources. Affluent patients who wished to pay for treatment generally were sent to the Toronto aslyum.[154] Of those who were admitted to London, a small proportion were found by the bursar to have some means of paying for their upkeep. In the absence of dependents, their assets were held in trust and administered by either the Inspector or a committee of relatives or friends. For those without resources, attempts were made to persuade the family to sign a bond for all or a negotiated portion of the weekly charge. The number of such paying patients never exceeded 15% of the total, and many fell into arrears[155] (Table 2.10). Yet the admission statistics show few individuals with no occupation, and male height and weight statistics suggest no gross nutritional deficiencies such as would be associated with extreme poverty.[156] The inability to pay was, then, not a reflection of pauperism, but of an economic category best described as working poor. A typical case illustrating this fragile economic status is that of a patient admitted in 1882, at which time a weekly

Table 2.10. *London Asylum expenditures and income from pay patients, selected years*

Year	Expenditure	Income	Income as percentage of expenditure
1878	87,394.84	7,317.37	8.4
1888	122,692.56	10,941.06	8.9
1898	137,201.95	12,166.50	8.9

Sources: IR, 1878, 24; 1888, 33; 1898, 20, 35.

sum of $2.75 was pledged. Upon discharge nine years later, the patient was in arrears by almost $1,300. The explanation of this default, in all likelihood, lies in the fact that the weekly charge represented one or two days wages for an unskilled farm or general laborer.[157] As a result, in 1886, for example, though patients technically designated as paying compromised over 13% of the asylum population, they contributed less than 10% of the total cost of patient maintenance.[158] The remaining 87% of patients were simply too poor for authorities even to entertain the expectation of payment.

The correspondence of the Inspector contains vivid testimony to the marginal economic circumstances of the London Asylum's clientele. On occasion, families were found to be "covering up property" belonging to the insane individual, while in other instances, though able, they simply refused to contribute toward the upkeep of a relative.[159] More often, however, even modest amounts exceeded the family's financial competence. John E., for example, signed a bond with an "X" in 1880 and paid $1.00 weekly for over a year before requesting that his wife be given free treatment. His farm was worth less than $2,000, was mortgaged for $1000, and from it he supported an aged mother and four children under the age of eleven. His promissory note was canceled, but other debtors were less fortunate.[160] The family of Margaret M. paid $1.50 per week for six months and then succeeded in reducing payments to $0.75. Her husband died leaving a farm worth, with chattels, $3,000 but encumbered by debts of $900. The remaining family consisted of four boys and three girls, all consumptives, who were able to do only the lightest work. The "family are industrious and even courageous in trying to make a living," wrote the Inspector, but, "two children have died, and the funeral expenses of these two and their father is [sic] not yet paid." Despite the "pathetic and touching" case, the Provincial Secretary refused to cancel the bond.[161] An equally piteous case was that of John B., and the concern he expressed for his child, born to his wife while she was an asylum patient. Having lost his land grant, he wrote from Northern Ontario in January, begging Bucke to care for the child until spring:

My wages just averages 10 dollars per month with Board. Men is plenty & work is rather scarce and when I support my three sons I takes me very busy. in summer I get better wages.[162]

Barely literate, scraping a living from casual labor, and caring alone for a family, John B. joined a great many other laboring poor in consigning family members to the care of the asylum. If committal gave acceptable shelter to the stricken relative, it also, as in the case of attendants, represented a strategy, a means of coping with economic adversity that gave at least temporary respite to the family. Poverty, then, became the significant distinguishing characteristic of the London institution's patients.[163]

When the patient arrived at the asylum, accompanied by the appropriate certificates, the diagnosis of insanity had already been made: It simply remained to classify the case, not according to diagnosis, but rather by level of cooperation. The "quiet chronic cases" were assigned to three cottages, each housing 60 patients, which stood apart from the main building. The cost of their operation was less than elsewhere in the asylum, largely because, according to Bucke, few attendants were required. If these buildings provided "bright and homelike" accommodation, residence there signified, in the Inspector's view, patients "past all hope of cure."[164] At the opposite end of the behavioral spectrum were the 186 cases assigned, after 1879, to another segregated building, the refractory ward. It housed "the very violent, the very dirty, and those who are determined to elope."[165] The walls were made of cement rather than plaster, the floors of hardwood, the ventilating apparatus of India rubber instead of earthenware, and the screened windows secured by external bars.[166] For the first years of operation, this ward revealed "neither good order nor neatness" and "in some parts of the building want of cleanliness was observable."[167] By 1883, with the introduction of work for the patients and the diminished use of mechanical restraint, the "scene of violence and mad confusion," so offensive to the Inspector, had become tranquil and orderly.[168] It remained, however, both the place of incarceration for patients perceived as violent as well as a means of coercion for uncooperative and rebellious individuals.

Patients who fell between the two extremes of chronic or incorrigible, more than 600 cases by the 1890s, were lodged in the vast main building. Here the wards were segregated by sex, as was the dining room, with little obvious attempt to group patients by age or diagnosis.[169] A daily routine, like the repetitive carbohydrate-laden menu, shaped the lives of the patients. Breakfast was served at 6:30 during the summer, and work commenced at 8:00, though in winter the entire schedule began an hour later. The lunch break occurred at 11:30, with a return to work following, between 1:00 and 4:30. After the meal, particularly during the winter, entertainments and dances were held in the dining hall.[170] Little overt restraint was employed, the patients instead finding themselves confined by a rigid schedule dominated by the imperative of assigned domestic or agricultural duties. Though the Superintendent and his assistant physicians were doubtless known to the patients, contact was brief and superficial. Instead, the attendants had charge of administering the patients' routine and, in all probability, of interpreting patients and physicians, accurately or otherwise, to each other. Such was the formal ward routine.

On a more covert level, ward life was by no means as routine as official views suggested. It is clear that the medical staff frequently had little detailed knowledge of the patients, either on initial contact when previous admissions to the same or other asylums were often unknown,[171] or later on the wards. In 1883, for example, a patient was found by his family, after discharge, to have a broken arm. Not only did the several asylum physicians disagree among themselves as to whether the arm was injured in the institution, but, as Inspector O'Reilly wrote, "The most unsatisfactory part of this case is . . . that it had not been noticed either by the attendants or by the medical officers, two of whom are supposed to have examined him."[172] As a result of the inability of four physicians to supervise adequately the daily affairs of 1000 inmates, the patients were left to the mercy of their attendants. Their authority was doubtless exerted through an unofficial system of privileges awarded or punishments allotted, a ritual common to many forms of institution life.[173] Inevitably, this pattern of negotiated interaction broke down and the attendants responded to recalcitrant patients with varying degrees of neglect or violence. On occasion, the consequences were sufficiently marked to draw the attention of the asylum hierarchy. A patient was scalded to death in a bath due to the inattention of an attendant. A female patient was sexually assaulted by a male attendant, "so brutish in nature" as to provoke Inspector Langmuir's surprise that such a man was employed at the asylum. An elderly patient sustained a fractured arm when struck with a stick by an attendant who claimed that "he attacked me and I had to defend myself."[174] Such incidents were, in fact, sufficiently common that the Inspector demanded the chief attendants record daily all "flesh wounds or discolouration" which then were to be examined by the physicians.[175] Despite this vigilance, the vast majority of "scratched and discoloured faces," the Inspector conceded, "on inquiry, were shown to be acts of patients or of those having the marks themselves."[176] The coercive aspects of the attendant–patient relationship remained to asylum officials elusive and seldom documented.

Though their opinions were often of little influence, patients and their families were by no means passive in their response to asylum treatment. Family members wrote to demand the release or transfer of their relatives, or to request a second opinion when faced with an unfavorable prognosis.[177] Such appeals coming from members of the external community were dealt with according to the circumstance of the individual case. Far more problematic were entreaties originating directly from the patients. These letters were often rambling, semiliterate accounts complaining of poor food, negligent attendants, or inappropriate incarceration. An engraged patient, for example, complained to Inspector Christie of his mistreatment by "a gang of Hypnotic Thugs . . . in the pay of this institution." If letters to the Inspector of this type were signed, Bucke was advised of the charges and, often, as in the above case, dismissed them as "fantasies."[178] In fact, he admitted in a similar case, generally "We do not . . . send these letters . . . I do not know how he got this one to the

Table 2.11. *Asylum admissions and discharges, selected years*

	Admitted		Discharged				
Year	Warrant	Certificate	Recovered	Improved	Unimproved	Died	Escaped
1878	73	141	47	17	6	42	4
1888	53	64	21	15	4	39	1
1898	25	107	50	17	4	48	3

Source: ARMS, 1878, 318; 1888, 41; 1898, 89.

post."[179] In effect, the institutionalization of the patient, signifying a deranged mind, was officially assumed to preclude the ability to lodge legitimate grievance against the asylum and its officials. In the case of an anonymous letter, when the author could not be clearly identified as a patient, the charges were disregarded on another basis. "I have little faith in such communications," wrote the Inspector, "and invariably presume there is some sinister motive operating."[180] Without confirmation by a community-based spokesman, complaints by patients were generally dismissed as little more than the aberrations of a disturbed mind. More animated protest, in all probability, would simply have served to confirm the patient's diagnosis.

Just as there were several modes of entry to the asylum, so the patients might take their leave by various routes. Least common were escapes. Typically, a male patient in the twenty-to-fifty age group simply wandered away from the asylum grounds, only to be returned within a week. Little detection was required since most went directly to their homes and were quietly apprehended by relatives and police. Only infrequently were escapees not recovered and were then written off as permanently "eloped."[181] Each year, 6 or 7% of the patients were sent out on probation. During most years, less than one-fifth of these were returned to the asylum and over one-third were declared recovered.[182] Warrant cases were not eligible for parole and, on occasion, relatives refused to accept responsibility for a patient for whom probation was suggested.[183] Between 4 and 7% of the patients were discharged yearly, most as recovered, a significant number as improved, and very few as unimproved (Table 2.11). It was a convention among alienists to calculate the number discharged as a percentage of the number admitted, with 45% considered high, and under 40% regarded as low.[184] Computed in this manner, Bucke's discharge rate in 1878 was 33%, in 1888 34%, and in 1898, 54%. For a portion of the patients, not a great deal fewer than were discharged yearly, only their demise removed them from the asylum. In 1878, discharges liberated 10% of the patients, while death occurred in 6% of cases. In 1888, the figure of 4% applied to both categories, and in 1898 the rates were 7% and 5%, respectively.[185] The most common cause of death was *senile decay*, followed closely by a similar condition, *marasmus*, a gradual wasting for no obvious reason. The other most frequently cited causes were tuberculosis, epilepsy, and apoplexy, though diagnoses were often vague and imprecise. As the causes suggest, patients over sixty, though few in number, accounted for a large proportion of the deaths. In 1890, for example, despite representing only 7% of the asylum population, they accounted for one-third of the deaths, while a decade later, though their numbers had increased to 12% within the institution, they comprised 58% of deaths.[186] Indeed, for the elderly, death appears to have been the common alternative to chronic residence in the institution. Exit from the London Asylum, then, was secured infrequently by escape, more commonly by parole, and most often by discharge or death.

The London Asylum, an imposing edifice of apparent authority and purpose, concealed a complex pattern of human relationships and ambiguous motivations.[187] To the provincial government, it was a means by which to deal with the debilitated poor in a manner suggesting beneficence. Such obvious concern for the destitute confirmed the legitimacy and, indeed, the largesse, of the existing political authority and the economic context in which it operated. To the government's discomfiture, the expense and size of the asylum rapidly escalated, despite the gospel of cost containment and efficiency propagated by vigilant Inspectors. This administrative perspective became the primary focus of the Medical Superintendent, gradually displacing his previous medical identity. Though he valued the financial security and social prestige associated with his post, the Superintendent was also subject to the same monotonous institutional routines as were the patients. It was one of the few characteristics which the medical staff shared with the attendants. To these (often ostensibly ill-qualified) employees was delegated, paradoxically, the important task of intimate daily contact with the patient population. It was an awkward role, for while the attendants shared a common social background and institutional routine with their charges, they were expected to function with authority and discipline. The attendants themselves doubtless viewed the asylum posts as an uncongenial and temporary shelter against economic adversity, rather than the selfless calling envisaged by the institutional hierarchy. The tension inherent in their ambiguous identity occasionally erupted in violence, shattering the outward order of asylum life to reveal brief glimpses of a harsher reality. It was this inner world, in addition to the overt institutional rules and regulations, that governed the quality of patient existence. Most inmates were from the lower depths of the working poor, debilitated individuals whose families could no longer cope – not with violence and disorder, but simply with peculiar and unproductive behavior. Many arrived hoping for little more than regular food and clean accommodation. For those families or patients sufficiently impressed by the physical size and medical authority of the asylum to entertain hope of cure, the reality must have come as a shocking disappointment. Chronicity was the rule, death not infrequent, and recovery distinctly uncommon. Indeed, in the final analysis, the asylum was a custodial institution not only for patients, but for a complex melange of other individuals and their ambiguous roles, identities, and expectations.

3

Toward a secular physiology of mind

Cloistered in the asylum, much of Richard M. Bucke's intellectual activity was directed toward formulating an understanding of the human mind. In this process he drew on his antecedent intellectual career which, from adolescence to the publication of his first book in 1879, was a microcosm of Victorian biomedical thought. As historians such as Frank Turner and L.S. Jacyna have cogently argued, the post-Darwinian conflict between science and religion was, in an important sense, a dispute between clerics and laypersons over the social applicability and authority of two types of knowledge.[1] This epistemological controversy, in effect, juxtaposed an older theological tradition convinced that the observational study of natural history revealed divine intent, against the secular conviction that empirical investigation alone could discover valid natural principles. Though lay scientists often argued that the results of their empiricism in no way challenged notions of design, their methodological contrast with the exponents of natural history created an intellectual watershed in Victorian science. It was a dispute from which, by the late 1870s, the professional lay scientists emerged largely victorious; never again would talented amateurs constitute themselves the cutting edge of British science.

In an analogous fashion Bucke himself moved from the childhood orthodoxy of his Church of England heritage to the latitudinarian comfort of Universalism. It proved a brief waystop on his journey to what he later referred to as *philosophical atheism*. Bucke's drift toward this position was enhanced while at medical school by his study of the vital force animating human life. It was, he concluded, a form of energy identical to the physical and chemical forces of the inorganic world and required no reference to any divinely conferred quality. These notions he found confirmed in the scientific doctrines of the Comtean positivism he encountered during postgraduate studies in London and Paris. In his journey toward the secularization of his cosmology Bucke was unable to rid himself of metaphysical notions that were increasingly anachronistic in the world of medical science. Yet both his methodology and the vocabulary in which he couched his work clearly derived from the secular impulse in physiology. In this manner he paralleled the route taken by many of his medical colleagues. Their view of physiology, and particularly the physiology of mind, abandoned a theological or metaphysical authority and turned instead to a secular legitimation rooted in the value-transcendent empiricism of biomedical science itself.

Aside from tutelage in his father's voluminous library as youth, Bucke had received no formal schooling until he entered McGill in 1858. Yet he was familiar with many of the intellectual issues of his day, particularly, as indicated by his childhood speculations, with theological debates. This suspicion is confirmed by his matriculation entry at medical school. There he listed his religion as Universalist, rather than the Church of England in which he had been raised, suggesting a deliberate conversion. It is possible that he chose this denomination as compatible with both his own free thought and with respectable entry to McGill, though other matriculants periodically recorded no religion at all.[2] But existing evidence suggests that he had some knowledge of and affinities to Universalist doctrines. The village to which the Bucke family emigrated was the center of upper Canadian Universalism. The Universalists had no hesitation in issuing public pronouncements on subjects such as temperance and capital punishment, or staging well-advertised debates between their spokesmen and more orthodox theologians. Though the Bucke family had every opportunity to learn of the sect, the 1842 census lists the family's affiliation as Church of England, a designation used by two of Bucke's older brothers when matriculating at McGill in the early 1850s.[3] It appears that Bucke's own affinity with Universalist doctrine derived from a later period, perhaps as a result of encounters with the aggressive Universalist missionaries who pushed through the American Midwest to California in the 1840s. A much more direct link between Bucke and the Universalists, however, grew out of his friendship with his prospecting partners, the Grosh brothers, and his subsequent close ties to their father, Aaron B. Grosh. The latter was a leader of American Universalism and maintained correspondence with Bucke until shortly before his death in 1884.[4] His letters to Bucke covered a range of topics, particularly the litigation involving his sons' mining claims, but most contained both religious advice and indications of close personal ties. If, during the 1860s, Bucke passed through a vehemently anti-clerical stage, his scorn was largely directed toward more conventional churches.

By 1858, in any case, Bucke found himself sufficiently comfortable with Universalism to accept its denominational designation at McGill. Its theology certainly imposed few doctrinal restrictions on a young man inclined toward free thought and, in fact, gave scope to a range of spiritual and social beliefs unacceptable to more orthodox Protestant churches.[5] With a seemingly nonchalant disregard for traditional views of an afterlife and an outright repudiation of the Trinity, the Universalists struck a marked contrast to the mainstream of Protestantism in the early nineteenth century.[6] In fact, puzzled theologians within the church joined critics from without in debating whether Universalism was, in fact, a branch of Christianity.[7] The Universalist doctrine of ultimate redemption for all and the hope that this belief would constitute a new world religion were similar to the themes upon which Bucke would base his best-known work, *Cosmic Consciousness* (1901). Universalists were animated by a supremely optimistic view of human potential, a perspective that led some (Bucke passively among them) to socialism and many to the conviction that their denomination was the religion most suited to the American style of democracy and republicanism. The strong emphasis on egalitarianism was a reflection of the predominantly working-class and agrarian support enjoyed by the Universalist Church, a constituency familiar to Bucke from his American rambles and celebrated in the Whitman poems he later found so appealing.[8] Nor did the church's doctrine prove incompatible with the science Bucke was soon to absorb. Universalism easily accepted Darwin's theories and one prominent member argued that Comte and Spencer were Universalists in all but name.[9] Equally, if science was accommodated by the church, so too was a strong affinity with spiritualism. Other denominations might view experiences such as Bucke's 1872 illumination with reserve, but Universalist theology traditionally harbored a strong mystical impulse.[10] Such affinities between Universalism and Bucke's later thought indicate that his early religious experience played a larger role in his intellectual development than even he might have been aware.

Yet in strictly denominational terms, it was an ephemeral role, for within half a decade he was to confess, in his diary, that he had become an atheist. That he was assisted in this transition by his medical studies is evident from his graduation thesis on "The Correlation of the Vital and Physical Forces." While he conceded that his subject was "not strictly a medical one," he felt that it dealt with "the nature of life" and, consequently, lay "at the basis of all branches of medicine." Bucke was quite correct in his assessment: The topic had bedeviled medical theory at least since the popularization of Cartesian dualism. The fundamental concern of such discussions was to identify the distinguishing feature of animate existence, to devise, in other words, a philosophically and physiologically congruent definition of life itself. The central task for participants in this debate was to ascertain the degree to which man could be understood as an autonomous physiological entity without reference to the direct creative intervention of God. Descartes had proposed one approach to this inquiry by banishing the soul from the legitimate domain of medicine and focusing instead on corporeal man, a clocklike machine no more complex than the sum of its constituent parts. At the opposite end of the early eighteenth-century interpretative spectrum, George Ernst Stahl argued that the human body transcended the inherent chemical and mechanical capacities of its components, a phenomenon explicable only by the invocation of a supra-added *anima* or life force of divine origin.[11] The parameters of the mechanist–vitalist debate had now been sketched; for a century and a half medical theorists, often highly eclectic and inconsistent, arranged themselves along a hazy continuum defined by this polarity.[12]

Though the volume of publication and the variety of viewpoints chosen seemed endless, disputants were engaged in a common cause.[13] How was it, they asked, that the living body, if no more than a collage of common chemicals, was seemingly able to disregard normal physical laws and resist the decay to which at death it immediately fell victim? Clearly a principle, not unlike

Newton's gravity in its pervasive applicability to natural phenomenon, would satisfy either side in the debate. What remained at issue, however, was whether this principle was inherent in the physical arrangement of the body or constituted a special, supra-added force.[14] By the 1830s British and European physiologists had reached a point of biomedical agnosticism. The slow accretion of experimental data gradually outweighed the credibility of a doctrine of supra-added vital force. Lavoisier's work on respiration and animal heat, Wohler's synthesis of the organic substance urea, and Schwann's elaboration of cell theory were events each of which challenged significant aspects of the vitalist tradition.[15] In fact, after the appearance of John Pritchard's critical *Review of the Doctrine of the Vital Principle* in 1829 and, seven years later, the third edition of John Bostock's *Elements of General Physiology,* references to a supra-added vital spirit became infrequent.[16] Taken together such studies seemed to have, on the one hand, discredited the concept by 1840, yet on the other, left nothing but a sceptical methodology in its place.

The 1840s proved a significant decade for both those physiologists who sought a unifying life principle and for those who demanded a rigid adherence to physical–chemical laws. To their mutual satisfaction, vitalists and materialists discovered a compromise in a newly refined doctrine of force. The technical conceptualization and vocabulary necessary to comprehend force occurred against a background of three important intellectual currents. The first was the tendency of German Romanticism to posit, in Thomas Kuhn's phrase, "a single unifying principle for all natural phenomena." Second, as George Rosen has argued, a "secular quantitative approach," derived from both factory economics and business accounting, spilled into scientific discourse and added credence to attempts to equate and balance energy production. Finally, a vague notion of the convertibility of force had been implicit in British natural history literature since the end of the eighteenth century.[17] Within this social and scientific context a dozen investigators during the 1840s groped their way toward the concept of the conservation of energy. Although most were engineers, at least three – Julius Mayer, Hermann Von Helmholtz, and Justus Liebig – were principally concerned with biological phenomena.

These various currents in physical science were synthesized and popularized by W.R. Grove in his lecture series, "On the Correlation of Physical Forces." He declared that "heat, light, electricity, magneticism, chemical affinity, and motion . . . may produce, or be convertible into, any of the others" and none could "originate otherwise than from some pre-existing force." His suggestion that the concepts of correlation and conservation of force, "might be applied to the organic as well as the inorganic world" fell on receptive ears.[18] Already, in 1837, the English physiologist, W.B. Carpenter, had declared that there was "nothing essentially different" in the laws regulating animate and inanimate creation.[19] Grove's lectures encouraged him to extend his arguments in his paper at the Royal Society in 1850, entitled, "On the Mutual Relations of the Vital and Physical Forces." It was here that the correlation doctrine received its most concise biological statement. Drawing on sources which included Schwann's well-known cell theory and Liebig's chemistry, Carpenter summarized his arguments in these terms:

Starting with the abstract notion of Force, as emanating at once from Divine Will, we might say that this force, operating through inorganic matter, manifests itself in electricity, magnetism, light, heat, chemical affinity, and mechanical motion but that, when directed through organized structures, it effects the operations of growth, development, chemico–vital transformation, and the like; and is further metamorphosed, through the instrumentality of the structures thus generated, into nervous energy and muscular power.[20]

In this formulation vital force, albeit of divine origin, had been reduced to simple physical–chemical interactions. It was this contention, borrowed from Grove and particularly Carpenter, upon which Maurice Bucke based his graduation thesis. Though he, too, paid lip service to a Divinity, it was a form of physiology in which such an outside agency was largely extraneous. Physiological discourse, in effect, was on the verge of complete secularization.

Bucke began his discussion of vital force with a brief historical review, culled directly from Carpenter's paper, in which he distinguished his physical–chemical conception of vitalism from the purely metaphysical versions of Stahl or Cullen. Most authorities, he continued, would agree that the elements constituting organic and inorganic creation differed in proportion rather than type and that the chemical forces binding these elements were likewise similar. In his thesis, however, he disputed the traditional notion that the forces operating in the material and in the living world were separated "by a well marked line." On the contrary, Bucke argued, "the forces we see manifested by organized beings are another and modified form of the forms existing in the inorganic world, borrowed from it, and when used again returned to it."[21] His definition of this process, illustrated by the example of the oxidation of zinc in a galvanic battery, was taken almost verbatim from Carpenter, while his discussion of the allied concept of conservation of force he based in large part on Henry Thomas Buckle's discussion of Faraday's work. Citing Grove's lectures, he took for granted that his readers would accept "as proved" the correlation of the various physical forces and, instead, turned his own attention to the relationship between the several forms of vital force.[22]

"All the forces . . . which are manifested by organized beings," Bucke wrote, "are evolved through the instrumentality of cells." Physical forces induce chemical changes within cells, which result in the liberation of chemical force. Depending on the character of the cell in which the reaction occurs, the chemical energy is manifested as one of a variety of vital forces. Ultimately, however, these assorted forces are correlated to each other and may be viewed as simply as one entity, *cell force*.[23] Most convincing was the case of nerve force, a form of energy similar but not identical to electricity, which appeared to be the highest form of vital force. Nerve force could be derived from body heat, from light falling on the retina, or from the mechanical irritation of nerve endings. Conversely, it was known to contribute to the generation of animal temperature, could, in the case of certain forms of marine life, produce luminosity, and it provoked the mechanical action of muscle contraction. For Bucke, as for Carpenter from whom he borrowed most of his arguments, the vital forces were clearly interchangeable forms of biological energy.[24]

Bucke had, then, established that physical forces were mutually convertible and, separately, that vital forces were correlated among themselves. It remained to demonstrate a point of intersection between these two systems in order to establish their ultimate unity as part of a larger whole. This Bucke attempted to do on two grounds, both arguments advanced by Carpenter in slightly different form. Plants, he first contended, transform simple chemical elements into more complex organic compounds. The newly formed molecules are chemically less stable than simple elements and require energy, provided by light and heat, to bind them in their vegetable form. These plants are then ingested by animals and broken down again into simple elements, in the process releasing their stored energy. This energy, which began as sunlight, is then transformed within cells into various forms of vital energy.[25] In his second argument, Bucke circumvented the vegetable world entirely, asserting instead that light and heat were known, at least in the case of coldblooded animals, to promote directly vital functions such as respiration, reproduction, and growth.[26] On the basis of these complementary lines of reasoning, Bucke felt he had adequately shown the link between physical and vital forces. Inorganic, vegetable, and animal matter became three discrete but closely knit aspects of a whole. If the system was initially "planned and formed by a Mind and Hand so infinitely superior in wisdom and power to those that work among us," it required no knowledge of or, indeed, belief in, that mastermind to thoroughly comprehend human physiology.[27]

Bucke's thesis, awarded the annual McGill prize and published in a Montreal medical journal, was clearly relevant to a major issue in midcentury physiology. It was, however, a rapidly disappearing focus of debate. A decade later, Osler's prize-winning graduation essay, "accompanied by 33 microscopic and other preparations of morbid structure," reflected the changes that were overtaking English physiology.[28] The traditional British preference for anatomical investigation rather than experimental studies found diminished space after 1870 in the new laboratories of Edward Shafer, Michael Foster, and John Burdon Sanderson.[29] Even more anachronistic was the metaphysical speculation associated with discussions of vitalism in which, as a "philosophic physiologist," Carpenter had been pleased to participate.[30] Claude Bernard's introduction of the concept of *internal environment* sealed the fate of the vitalist tradition. If, within organisms, there were processes unfamiliar in the field of inorganic chemistry, these processes Bernard established were not necessarily inexplicable in terms of the same basic principles that applied to the inorganic world.[31] Victorian physicians, in effect, adopted a new mode of perceiving the body. Far from representing the pinnacle of divine creation, the functions of which could be inferred from its mechanical parts, the body was now viewed as simply the sum of familiar physiochemical reactions. It was a physiological paradigm the unity of which derived not from the intent of an immanent God, but from an entirely secular system of natural principles. These changes – the secularization of physiology – left Bucke in an oddly transitional position. His thesis clearly pointed toward the materialist physiology of the 1870s, while his methodology and style of argument were rooted in an older, and largely metaphysical tradition.

During the three years that followed his graduation from medical school, Bucke's diaries portray him as a voracious reader. Encouraged by his English friends, Alfred and Henry Forman, he pursued French, English, and German fiction, and developed a particular affinity for the English romantic poets. The most important interest that Bucke shared with the Forman brothers, however, was not literature but positivism. He first learned of this philosophy in the fall of 1862 by reading G.H. Lewes's *Biographical History of Philosophy* (1845). At the time, he was visiting his relatives at Milden Hall in Norfolk. He found their orthodox religious and social views oppressive and it seems unlikely that his copy of Lewes came from their library.[32] In all probability it was one of the Formans who recommended the work to Bucke. Harry was a contributor to the *Fortnightly Review* (often assumed at the time to represent a positivist viewpoint), and an acquaintance of George Eliot, one of Comte's English sympathizers.[33] To Bucke he wrote of the "fierce pleasure" he derived from the French philosopher, and closed at least one of his letters with the phrase, "in the name of Comte." His correspondence often contained lengthy discussions of English positivism and lamentations on the difficulty of having such views accepted in a conservative society. Alfred was at first an equally spirited follower of positivism, echoing Harry by signing a letter to Bucke, "Your Affectionate Brother in Comte." His enthusiasm gradually dissipated and, after a flirtation with Schopenhauer's theories, he decided in 1875 to disavow all philosophical systems.[34] During Bucke's sojourn in England, however, Harry and Alfred were both ardent positivists.

It is unlikely that Bucke required any persuasion to accept Comte's major tenets, though it was not until he had been in

Paris some months that his French was sufficiently agile to approach with confidence the philosopher's original works. Even before reading this material he recalled preaching "the principle of positivism and philosophical atheism" to a bewildered fellow student in England. This early enthusiasm may have been fostered, as well, by Benjamin Ward Richardson who, during the 1850s, shared his London home with one of Comte's leading English followers. Positivism was also a system of thought endorsed by Bucke's teacher at University College, Russell Reynolds, whose *System of Medicine* he later found indispensable.[35] Ensconced in Paris, in April 1863, he read Emile Littré's *Paroles de Philosophie Positive* (1858) which he enjoyed, and shortly after began *Catéchisme Positiviste* (1852). This work he found more difficult but four weeks later declared it "one of the loveliest books in existence." By the fall of that year he wrote in his diary that "as I come to know still more of Comte I shall go with him still further" since he is "the greatest mind that I have ever come in contact with." He began to read Comte's work two hours each day, likely starting with *Système de Politique Positive* (1851–4), which he had purchased in May. Three years later he still hoped to finish the four volumes but admitted, from past experience, "I am afraid I shall stick in it."[36] How much more of Comte's work Bucke ever read is uncertain. He did read commentaries on the French philosopher such as that contained in John Stuart Mill's *Logic* or in his essay in the *Westminister Review* for 1865.[37] He preferred Comte to either Mill or Herbert Spencer and as late as 1867 attempted, with little success, to make detailed notes on Comte's six-volume *Cours de Philosophie Positive* (1830–2).[38] In a letter to Harry Forman in 1870 he referred to Comte as "the Great Master" and quoted him, nine years later, in an introductory epigraph to his first book.[39] Positivism, it seems reasonable to conclude, made a substantial impact on Bucke's thought in the 1860s, an impact that would reverberate throughout his later published work.

Why, in 1863, did positivism provide at least a partial answer to what Bucke referred to as his "unappeasable hunger for enlightenment"? As he pored over G.H. Lewes's estimate of Comte, a book to which he felt himself "forever indebted," he would have learned of the prevailing "anarchy in the higher regions" of European thought. It was a chaos born of philosophy's "centuries of failure," of the metaphysician's unrequited search for certitude. Disillusioned, thoughtful men "withdrew themselves more and more from Philosophy, and devoted their speculative energy to science." Unfortunately, entrenched in their own narrow specialties, scientists proved ill-suited to the "construction of general doctrines." At this critical juncture Auguste Comte introduced a philosophical system that was both rigorous in its application of scientific method and all-encompassing in its scope. In fact, Bucke would have learned, Comte discussed and classified in a hierarchy all branches of human knowledge, placing the physician's interest, biology, second only to sociology. In their maturation, each of these disciplines mirrored the upward evolution of human society through successive stages, the theological, the metaphysical, and, finally, the scientific. This evolutionary doctrine with its strong anticlerical ring, especially in the oppressively orthodox Victorian household in which he read Lewes's book, must have come as a refreshing message to Bucke. Even more intriguing was Lewes's insistence that Comte accomplished his philosophical goals without indulging in idle speculation as to first causes. This was in marked contrast, for example, to "the metaphysical physiologist" who "guesses" at "what he calls a 'vital principle' " and "pronounces it 'electricity' or 'nervous fluid', or 'chemical affinity'."[40] The reference to the materialist defeat of vitalism alone must have been sufficient to spark Bucke's further interest. Certainly, as Lewes noted in another work, the doctrine of Comte was best calculated to find "acceptance among those men of science whose preliminary studies in some sort qualify them to receive it – namely, the physiologists."[41] In this judgment he was substantially correct. Comte's leading disciples, Emile Littré in France and Richard Congreve in England, were both physicians, and medical men formed a large occupational category among known members of positivist groups. Maurice Bucke, in effect, joined a sizeable number of his professional colleagues in his affinity for positivism. The empirical precepts of a secular medical science not only banished theological rivals from the study of the natural world, but also provided the promise of a foundation from which that new science could be elaborated into a science of society. The doctrines of positivism, in short, promised nothing less than a justification for the social authority to which more than a few physicians of the period aspired.[42]

Once in France, with Lewes's introduction to positivism fresh
in his memory, Bucke wasted little time in acquiring works by
or about Auguste Comte. From this reading he derived his
belief that in biological explanations lay the key to understanding philosophical problems. The purpose of his philosophy,
Comte had written, was to frame a synthesis, a unifying "system which shall comprehend human life under every aspect."[43]
All "inquiry into *causes* properly so called, first or final" were
dismissed as "essentially idle." Instead, the new synthesis was
based on the belief that the laws of natural science such as those
described by Kepler, Galileo, or Newton were applicable "to all
phenomenon, whatever, social and moral quite as much as simply material." Bucke himself, in his McGill thesis, had used
physics and chemistry to explain *nerve force,* though he had
stopped short of extending his analogy to mental processes, and
doubtless had little difficulty in accepting Comte's line of
reasoning. But the nature of human behavior and social relationships was not to be discerned through mathematical or
physical laws; rather, their elucidation depended on the relatively new science of biology. "Humanity being but the highest
degree of animality" Comte wrote, "the highest notions of sociology, and even of morals, have necessarily their first germs
in biology, for the really philosophical minds which can detect
them there."[44] It was, he continued, only in the nineteenth century that biology had developed sufficiently to provide a basis
for sociology. The thinkers to whom he acknowledged a conceptual debt were individuals from whom Bucke, too, would
borrow in his work on the sympathetic nervous system. The
"incomparable Bichat," Comte felt, first demonstrated that the
"simplest functions of life" obey the same laws as are operative
in the inorganic world, a viewpoint with which Bucke certainly
would have expressed no disagreement. Franz Joseph Gall, "by
an effort of genius," founded "the positive theory of human
nature." His accomplishment was to argue that the various
"higher functions" could be localized to specific areas of the
brain, that mind, in effect, was a function of the organization of
the human nervous system. A similar concern, the physical localization of man's moral sense, provided the focus for Bucke's
first book. Finally Cabanis, Comte felt, had demonstrated that
human cognition was ultimately based on sensory impression, a

view that corresponded to the associationist psychology that characterized British empiricism and upon which Bucke would base his own view of man's thought processes.[45] Biology, then, for both Comte and Bucke provided the key to understanding individuals and their social relationships.

A specific example of biology's explanatory utility, and a second significant area in which Bucke was influenced by Comte, concerned the nature of religion. By 1863, Bucke had passed from the paper-thin theism of Universalism to, as he put it, "philosophical atheism," a process perhaps not uncommon among members of such denominations.[46] Positivism claimed to furnish the requisite materials for a new secular faith, a claim to which Bucke's inherently religious if doctrinally skeptical temperament was openly receptive. "A sound theory of Biology," Comte argued, "furnishes the Positive theory of Religion with a foundation wholly unassailable." Man's mind, as sensualist psychology revealed, depended for its content on impressions gained from the external world, particularly from interaction with fellow beings. Seen in this light, each individual mind was but a small part of a collective human mentality or consciousness, which Comte labeled "the Great Being." Religion for Comte, then, in contrast to the "moral and political degradation of the theological priesthood," simply expressed "the state of perfect *unity*, which is distinctive of our existence." After death, the only immortality was the memory left by the soul in "the heart and mind of others."[47] This secularized religion was something of an embarassment to many of Comte's followers and they would have quietly assented to Lewes's suggestion that over his efforts "to become the founder of a new religion, let us draw the veil." Still others, however, such as Frederic Harrison or Richard Congreve found aspects of the new religion filled needs that orthodox doctrines did not.[48] It was with the latter group that Bucke was to side. Though his philosophy was to be reshaped in the 1870s so that "while being as a religion as positive as positivism it will supply more hope for mankind,"[49] his attitude toward religion bore a basic Comtean imprint.

The positivist theory of religion was founded on a biological conception of human nature. Fundamental to this viewpoint was the third major topic on which Comte influenced Bucke's thought, the relationship between mind and body. Already, as indicated by his McGill thesis, Bucke was willing to equate the vital forces, among them, "nerve force," with known physical or chemical forces. In Comte he found this materialistic impulse expanded to include the ultimate workings of the human mind. The "physical as well as the moral nature," Comte asserted, "are, in fact, so bound up together that no true harmony is possible if one tries to separate them." Specifically, Gall had shown that the mind, "the plurality of our higher functions," was a simple function of the brain. It was not, in contrast to the view of many metaphysicians, a supra-added soul unrelated to the corporal being.

The laws of logic by which the positivist brain functioned were clearly analogous to the physical laws by which the world itself operated. Nor did this materialistic interpretation apply to the intellect alone; it included the moral sense as well. Here Comte relied on the views of Bichat to assert that the "affective region" of the brain was linked only to "the chief organs of the life of nutrition." In effect, the moral nature, as Bucke was to argue as the basis of his first book, was localized to the abdominal viscera. The practical implication of this somatic view of morality was "to include health under religion, so as to make moral science, in its full conception, extend to medicine."[50] In his approach to mental illness, Bucke would rely heavily on a belief in somatic and psychic unity, a conviction he derived largely from his reading of Comte.

The essence of man's moral nature was of more than passing interest to Comte: In fact, it provided the underpinning for his theory of history. It was in this context that positivism exerted a fourth and final influence on Maurice Bucke. Traditional religions which "placed perfection in detachment from earth" were repugnant to Comte. Instead, he proposed that man's mind was evolving from an initial theological stage of superstition, through a transitional stage characterized by metaphysical abstractions, to a definitive era of scientific or positive truth. This final stage represented "that mastery which man alone can attain over all his defects, especially those of his moral nature." This "moral improvement" was a consequence of "the general laws of hereditary transmission" which were "even more applicable to our noblest attributes as to our lowest."[51] In his evolutionary perspective Comte owed less to Lamarck than he did to Bichat, Gall, and Saint-Simon.[52] Similarly, Bucke's view of history as a

chronicle of moral evolution was rooted less in Darwinian naturalism, though he clearly accepted such views, than in Comtean
positivism.[53] Significantly, this perspective would provide the
thesis for his most widely known work, *Cosmic Consciousness*
(1901).

To be a positivist in North America during the 1860s was to
belong to a diminutive and perhaps suspect group.[54] yet Bucke
was prepared to accept Comte's ideas in part on the basis of his
earlier exposure to both Universalist theology and to W.B. Carpenter's views on the physical nature of vital force. In a more
general sense, however, his positivist studies coincided with a
revolution in biological thought. Works such as those published
in the late 1850s by Virchow and Darwin combined to reveal an
entirely new way of viewing man and creation. The potential of
such innovative perspectives must have seemed, to many physicians, aptly captured in Comte's grandiloquent synthesis, with
the substantial role it assigned to biological knowledge. Comte
was hardly a consistent thinker and his prolix volumes, as one
frustrated scholar has commented, "are to the last degree invo-
luted, opaque, repetitious, in fact unreadable without an effort
almost as heroic as his devotion to writing them."[55] Moreover,
Bucke himself was not a systematic philosopher, and the concepts he borrowed from the chaotic French sage were never re-
integrated into a coherent, positivist whole. But Bucke did adopt
several major concepts from Comte's work, beliefs that, in effect, created the intellectual superstructure upon which all his
later work was based. Neither his reading of Darwin nor his
close association with Walt Whitman exerted a comparable influence. No source better prepared him to join many of his fellow
physicians in forging a secular epistemology with which to attack
the problem of mental physiology.

Bucke's participation in that assault did not begin until he had
completed several years of general practice. "I have no chance for
anything like regular study," he complained to Harry Forman in
1869, "and if I read a short article something is sure to occur
before the day is out to drive it all out of my head." Worse still,
as he lamented a year later, "I live here in a state of Egyptian
darkness as regards the light from the literary world. . . . There
is absolutely no one here that reads." Despite the constraints of
time and lack of stimulation, however, he admitted, "I am as full
of schemes for reading and studying all conceivable books and

subjects as ever." His correspondence with Forman testified to the accuracy of this assertion. In a typical letter, for example, his discussion of Herbert Spencer, G.H. Lewes, and Charles Darwin was followed by brief comments on the poetry of William Morris and Algernon Swinburne. Forman supplied Bucke with literary gossip and faithfully filled his orders for books, a task made none the easier by the diversity of titles requested. A letter from the winter of 1869, for instance, asked for a medical text by Russell Reynolds, the British pharmacopia, and works by Herbert Spencer, Thomas Carlyle, Charles Baudelaire, and Johann Goethe.[56] The hapless Forman may have shuddered at the catholicity of these requests but the titles were pedestrian in comparison to the esoteric works sought during Bucke's later fascination with Eastern religions. By way of consolation, he could rest secure in the knowledge that his letters to Bucke represented a literary lifeline to an intellect stranded in colonial isolation.

It was only after his mystical experience in England in 1872 that Bucke resolved to write a book on mental physiology, in which, he claimed, "he sought to embody the teaching of that illumination."[57] The work to which he referred, *Man's Moral Nature,* was based on a discussion of the functions of the sympathetic nervous system. It was a subject that, by its very complexity, invited speculative analyses. To Victorian physicians, the autonomic nervous system, charged with the control of involuntary bodily functions, was the least understood of the major components in the human nervous structure. Thomas Willis, writing in 1664, introduced the concept of involuntary movement and postulated that the system existed to coordinate such activities or, in the terminology of the period, "bring them into sympathy" with each other. It was a Danish anatomist, J.B. Winslow, who, in 1732, coined the term *great sympathetic nerve* and completed the description of the gross anatomy of the system, but the histological structure was to await elucidation until the mid-nineteenth century.[58] At that time an increasing number of independent physiological functions were assigned to these nerves. Ernst and Eduard Weber established the role of the vagus nerve in slowing the heart rate, in 1845, and Carl Ludwig demonstrated, several years later, that autonomic stimulation of the salivary glands increased secretion. A more general function was described by Claude Bernard and C.E. Brown-Séquard in 1851–

2 when they independently demonstrated aspects of the sympathetic control of regional blood flow.[59] By the 1870s, then, the gross and much of the microscopic anatomy of the sympathetic nerves was established and a number of physiological actions were ascribed to this system.

It was against this background that Bucke began his own consideration of the sympathetic nervous system. Though it was, he claimed, a subject about which he had thought in a general sense for many years, he recalled that he began "making notes on my speculations in moral philosophy or whatever you like to call it" in the fall of 1871 and later referred to this as the germinal period of his work. At that time he asked Forman to obtain from Benjamin Ward Richardson information "as to the Sympathetic System and its literature."[60] It was the latter's view, sent to Bucke ten weeks later, that "the most important book to be consulted is Davey on the Ganglionic nervous sytem," while "the basis of the whole inquiry is to be found in a much older work . . . Bichat's treatise on Life and Death." Certainly, in his own writing, Richardson echoed Bichat's general conclusions as to the function of the sympathetic system.[61] Forman was eventually able to provide a copy of Davey's book, but after reading it Bucke confided that he was quite "disappointed" in its contents. Similarly, he requested a new work by Edward Meryon, but on receipt wrote to Forman "I think it will help me a little but I doubt not much."[62] He also requested "a prize essay on the Great Sympathetic, written by two Germans . . . I think the prize was given by some French academy." There is no record of Forman locating this obscure reference.[63] Bucke continued to search for relevant sources, including in his later reading Henry Maudsley's *Physiology of Mind* (1876) and Russell Reynolds's essays on neurology in his *System of Medicine* (1870).[64] Despite the diligence of his neurological research, however, he found himself for several years unable to express his thoughts in written form.

His project progressed through several stages. In 1871 he explained his general intention to Henry Forman:

The thing has occupied my mind a great deal since I saw you and I am more and more impressed with the importance of it, but I almost despair of ever being able to put it into such shape as to make it assimilable for other minds. It is such a confounded big affair I don't feel as if I could handle it. It will be nothing less than a new theory of all art and religion and I am sure a true one. It will furnish a sound basis for poetical and other art criticism . . . It will supply a new theory of the universe and of man's relation to the external universe and while being as a religion as positive as positivism it will supply more hope for mankind and will not shut up men's faculties in the known and present in the same way that positivism does.[65]

Faced with a task of such magnitude, a year later he found he was unable "to put my ideas into intelligible shape" or "onto paper." In frustration he resolved, in 1875, to abandon a book and write, instead, a series of articles. He apparently succeeded in preparing a paper which he presented to a local medical society, though no copy of this work is extant.[66] Two years later the thesis of his speculations was presented at the annual meeting of the Association of Medical Superintendents of American Institutions for the Insane and, under the title "The Functions of the Great Sympathetic Nervous System," appeared in the *American Journal of Insanity*. This article Bucke considered "quite a success" and received qualified praise from Forman. The following year he elaborated on his theme in an essay published in the same journal, entitled, "The Moral Nature and the Great Sympathetic." He felt that in some quarters this article made "quite a furor," a reaction that hardened his resolve to incorporate his views into a book-length study.[67]

At first, in 1878, he found the writing of the book "a perfect nightmare,"[68] but gradually his intentions clarified. "I want the book to be published in a popular manner," he wrote to Forman,

It aught [sic] to be some such a book to the public as Richardson's 'Diseases of Modern Life' though scarcely so scientific and more popular. It will be a book for everyone to read but only thinkers and men with a spice of science about them will fully understand it . . .[69]

It was essential, in fact, that the book be written in popular form, for it was an "announcement of an immense and valuable discovery, affecting every man in the most vital manner." On the evening of November 19, 1878, he completed what he described to Forman as "a very remarkable and very valuable book."[70] (Figure 10.)

Figure 10. Title page and neurological illustrations from *Men's Moral Nature* (1879). Source: R. M. Bucke, *Man's Moral Nature* (New York: G. P. Putnam's Sons; Toronto: Willing and Williamson, 1879).

MAN'S

MORAL NATURE

AN ESSAY

BY

RICHARD MAURICE BUCKE, M.D.

MEDICAL SUPERINTENDENT OF THE ASYLUM FOR
THE INSANE, LONDON, ONTARIO

" I am a man who is preoccupied of his own soul."

NEW YORK
G. P. PUTNAM'S SONS
TORONTO, ONT.: WILLING & WILLIAMSON
1879

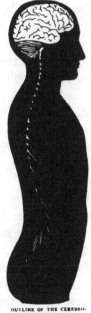

OUTLINE OF THE CEREBRO-
SPINAL NERVOUS SYSTEM.
Page 60.

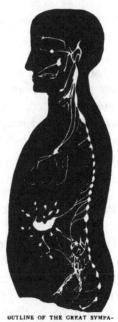

OUTLINE OF THE GREAT SYMPA-
THETIC NERVOUS SYSTEM,
Page 48.

With a dispassionate equanimity born of hindsight and passing time, Bucke later wrote of his book, *Man's Moral Nature,* "as was to be expected for many reasons . . . it had little circulation." This, indeed, was a far cry from his predictions following publication. Although he realized that all authors "think their first book will be a hit," he was convinced "people are scattered all over the States and Canada" who "are anxious to buy it."[71] Unfortunately, persuading an American publisher of the likelihood of such sales had proved a difficult task. Appleton, Scribner's, and several others turned the manuscript down sight unseen, informing Bucke that "a book called 'Man's Moral Nature' would not pay, no odds how able it was." Finally, G.P. Putnam agreed to accept the book if Bucke guaranteed costs of $700 to be recovered through the sale of 1000 copies. An arrangement under which Macmillan would publish simultaneously in Great Britain so as to secure Bucke's copyright proved abortive, and Forman was unable to find another firm.[72] "I don't think you need trouble yourself on the score of possible pirates," the ever-tactful Harry consoled, "for the book is a great deal too scientific to be a quick selling book enough to tempt them."[73] Eventually 25 copies were sent to Trubner and Company in England to be released under their imprint, but Forman's subtle prediction of meager sales proved accurate. Bucke at first felt the "book is being very well received here and is selling very fairly," but the actual figures must have changed his mind. Trubner sold 4 copies during the first year, while four years after publication, of the 750 copies produced, 241 had been sold in North America. Bucke purchased the remaining copies from Putnam in 1883, but it was another five years before he could bring himself to ask Forman to collect the unsold copies at Trubner's and "give them away if you can find anyone who will take them."[74]

The most obvious explanation for the book's lack of popular success was its abstruse subject matter and highly technical jargon. Yet both the vocabulary it employed and the neurological issues with which it dealt were very much a part of the medical environment of the 1870s. Indeed, Maurice Bucke began his neurological speculations during a period in which the functions of many areas of the nervous system were topics of vigorous academic discussion. Most authorities agreed, however, on the general theoretical postulate that specific neurological functions could be localized to separate areas of the nervous system, a consensus quite in contrast to the debates that characterized the early decades of the century.[75] It was Franz Joseph Gall, whose work Bucke had found celebrated by Comte, who had sparked the localization disputes by arguing that man possessed twenty-seven innate faculties, each situated in a specific region of the cerebral cortex.[76] Among his many critics, Pierre Flourens was the best known. Though he himself had localized several motor functions to areas of the brainstem or cerebellum, he denied that the higher psychic functions described by Gall could be isolated in the cerebral cortex and argued instead that the brain operated only as an integrated whole. This doctrine, compatible with the prevailing unitary view of higher functions and unassailable with the experimental techniques of the period, dominated medical thought into the 1840s.

Gall's intentions, however, were not forgotten. By midcentury, innovations in electrophysiology by investigators such as Emil Du Bois Reymond and Hermann von Helmholtz, as well as changing views of psychological mechanisms, prepared the ground for renewed attempts to localize cortical function. In fact, there had been a gradual accumulation of isolated but suggestive experimental evidence from Luigi Rolando's animal studies in 1809 to Gabriel Andral's careful clinical work in Paris during the 1830s. Such developments combined to give theoretical credibility to Paul Broca's well-known paper of 1861, which explained aphasia, the loss of speech without muscular paralysis, on the basis of a specific lesion in the third convolution of the frontal lobe. Less than a decade later Gustav Fritsch and Eduard Hitzig mapped the areas of the canine cortex that controlled muscular contractions of the face, neck, and limbs. Though the leading British physiologists, John Burdon Sanderson and Michael Foster, remained skeptical, the German work was confirmed during the 1870s by David Ferrier, E.A. Shafer, and Victor Horsely.[77] Cortical localization had become a physiological reality.

The new doctrine, it is important to emphasize, represented a significant departure from Gall's theories. The late-Victorian investigators rejected the phrenological attempt to isolate anatomically psychic functions such as love or self-esteem and, instead, spoke simply in terms of areas of motor action or sensory perception. Their interest, in effect, was with purely physiological categories while Gall's was primarily psychological.[78] Yet if cerebral physiology was, by the 1870s, a discipline quite distinct from psychology, it was, nevertheless, intimately connected to it. In particular, associationist psychology had grown up with neurological localization theory in an almost symbiotic fashion.[79] The basic assumptions of this approach to mental activities was hardly new to the nineteenth century. Rejecting innate ideas, John Locke had argued that thought represented combinations of elemental sensations derived entirely from experience. Many philosophers and physicians throughout the eighteenth century modified but did not abandon this basic premise, but it was a form of analysis that seemed progressively more tangential to the interests of medicine.[80] While Locke had taken his cue from Newtonian physics, by the middle of the nineteenth century this approach to psychology appeared little better than a division of metaphysics, with scant connection to biological or physical knowledge. Two currents in medical thought, however, revived interest in the relevance of associationist analysis. First, while rejecting Gall's concept of innate faculties, his view that the mind could be resolved into discrete functional subunits associationists found entirely compatible with their assumption that complex intellectual operations simply represented combinations of elementary mental functions. Secondly, the beginning with the work of Charles Bell and Francois Magendie, the basic functions of the nervous system were seen in terms of sensory perception and the initiation of motor activity, categories of conceptualization susceptible to measurement and quite distinct from older metaphysical categories such as the faculties suggested by Gall.[81]

This midcentury transformation in English psychology grew largely from the work of Alexander Bain and Herbert Spencer. Bain was labeled by Maurice Bucke as "a deuced clever writer" of "the orthodox opinion." By this description he may have meant that Bain's writing borrowed heavily from the associationist psychology of J.S. Mill, a philosopher whose work Bucke read and admired.[82] Perhaps reflecting his early interest in phrenology, in *The Senses and the Intellect* (1855) Bain retained the basic faculties of intellect, will, and feeling. These, however, he argued, could be resolved into associated components derived from sensation which, in turn, he conceived of in sensory–motor terms based largely on the work of the German physiologist Johannes Müller.

By utilizing a physiological definition of sensation, Bain believed he had removed his psychology from metaphysics and placed it with biology as an empirical science. Herbert Spencer, like Bain, paradoxically indebted to both Gall and Mill, also participated in the transformation of associationist psychology. Maurice Bucke read Spencer's *Social Statistics* (1852), written during a phrenological phase, with enthusiasm, though he felt his later *Principles of Psychology* (1855), was "undoubtedly damn poor stuff."[83] Yet he did not, as his own work would reveal, escape Spencer's influence. By arguing that sensation, as a physiological phenomenon, was identical from unicellular life to man, and by emphasizing that all sensation derived from interaction between the organism and the environment, Spencer adopted Bain's position that psychology was a biological science.[84] By the 1870s, then, explicitly metaphysical categories, whether innate or sensational, were banished from medical psychology to be replaced by simple sensory or motor operations as the building blocks of conscious thought. The analysis of mind would henceforth take place less in philosophical or theological discourse, than in a laboratory ruled by the dual orthodoxy of cerebral localization and associationist psychology.

It was against this conceptual background that Bucke's first book took shape. Its central focus was what he had learned from Comte was "the true and final science," a synthesis of both biology and sociology, that is, the study of man's moral nature. That the individual possessed an innate moral faculty was a conviction he had encountered in much of the contemporary psychological literature and particularly in Spencer's *Social Statics* (1852).[85] The specific purpose of his book, Bucke stated, was twofold: First, he intended to define the human moral sense and assign to it an anatomical location; secondly, he planned to determine whether this faculty was progressively reaching higher levels of development and, if so, for what reasons.[86] The method by which he attacked his objective had several general features borrowed from the sources with which he was familiar and employed according to the demands of his argument. First, as was the case in much of British physiology in the period before 1870,[87] he attempted to infer physiological function by observing anatomical form. The "cells and fibres of the great sympathetic system," he wrote, "differ materially in structure from the cells and fibres of the cerebro–spinal nervous system, and it can scarcely be supposed that such difference in structure should not be manifested by some corresponding difference in function." A similar methodological assumption appeared in Edward Meryon's 1872 study of the sympathetic system but, unlike Bucke, he was willing to cite extensive experimental literature.[88] This contrast pointed to the second significant feature of Bucke's approach: a rejection of the applicability of experimental physiology. "I have quoted very few experiments," he explained, "for the reason that I put very little confidence in the deductions drawn from them. To divide large sympathetic trunks, or to remove large sympathetic ganglia, must cause a disturbance of the general system which would necessarily mask to a great extent the peculiar effects flowing from the lesion of the nerves operated on; and any one who has paid attention to the literature of this subject cannot have failed to notice how contradictory are the positions supposed to be established by these means."[89] Vivisection, in other words, produced artifact rather than verifiable knowledge. Bucke's final methodological characteristic was his use of deductive reasoning, a description, given his respect for Francis Bacon,[90] with which he would have been uncomfortable. Nonetheless, from three general principles – associational psychology, neurological localization, and human evolution – supported by an eclectic blend of historical and speculative evidence, he attempted to deduce a theory of the sympathetic nervous system.

Bucke began his study with a general analysis of human thought, an overview designed primarily to distinguish between the intellect and the moral sense, according primacy to the latter. The intellect he located in the cerebrum and assigned it the task of registering sensory perceptions in the memory, as well as making judgments and comparisons. The initial sensory impressions were converted by the intellect into simple ideas, such as that signifying a color or shape, and then combined to form more sophisticated conceptions in the processes of reasoning or imagination. In this description of the functions of intellect there was little that departed from conventional views as, for example, expressed by J.G. Davey in his work on the sympathetic system. Similarly, the association process was conceived in terms that differed little from accounts in sources such as W.B. Carpenter's physiology text, which Bucke had studied at McGill, Comte's

Systems of Positive Polity, or Alexander Bain's *The Senses and the Intellect.*[91] In contrast to this intellectual apparatus stood the other principle contributor to mentation, the moral nature, a "bundle of faculties," the most elementary of which were love, faith, hate, and fear. Like Bain, Bucke retained several basic faculties as innate characteristics, but then argued that the moral nature, in the same manner as the intellect, functioned by associating its primary elements into more complex combinations. A constant succession of emotional states and intellectual concepts "flow on side by side without interfering with one another," until such time as a specific emotion may spontaneously associate with a specific idea to form a compound structure. Human thought, then, was composed of simple concepts, elemental emotions, and various combinations of these units.[92] Though simplistic, Bucke was generally, as he had once observed of Alexander Bain, "of the orthodox opinion." Bain, for his part, thought Bucke's psychological analysis did "not exhaust the component parts" nor were his categories "precise in themselves."[93] Yet Bucke's view of mind hinted at the more unorthodox opinions that were to follow for he credited the moral nature, not the intellect as was generally done, with responsibility for man's progressive evolution from a state of animality.[94]

Having considered the general outlines of human thought, Bucke narrowed his focus to the functions of the sympathetic nervous system. Following conventional views, he described the sympathetic innervation of "unstriped muscle," the control of glandular secretion, and the regulation of digestion and blood flow. Though perhaps dissenting on matters of detail, few authorities would have quarreled up to this point with Bucke's general description of sympathetic functions.[95] But it was here that Bucke introduced his thesis, "a THOUGHT," which he had discovered "years ago," and had recognized immediately that it "contained what I had so long looked for."[96] Simply stated, the sympathetic nervous system was "the physical basis of the moral nature."[97] This viewpoint he doubtless found confirmed by Xavier Bichat, first during the 1860s when reading Comte's laudatory account of his work, and later by pursuing, at the suggestion of his friend Benjamin Ward Richardson, the French histologist's *Physiological Researches on Life and Death* (1809).[98] According to Bichat, "Numerous sympathetic relations unite all the internal viscera

with the brain," which then combine to express "our moral affec-
tions." Each of the major structures connected by the sympathetic
system, "sometimes the digestive organs, sometimes the circula-
tory system, and sometimes the viscera belonging to the secretions" exert their influence on our "passions."[99] Bichat's division
of human existence into an animal life mediated by the central
nervous system and an organic life served by the sympathetic
proved a popular dichotomy. Gradually the concept of organic life
was absorbed into the physiological descriptions of involuntary
vegetative functions and the emphasis on passions and emotions
quietly discarded. Davey, for example, argued in his study that
the sympathetic ganglia of the abdomen were the seat of life itself,
but life defined only in a physiological sense as the sum of secretion, nutrition, respiration, and digestion. Attaching a moral connotation to the sympathetic system had become, in the later nineteenth century, as implausible as the phrenologists' attempt to
localize discrete psychic faculties in the cerebrum. As the noted
English alienist Daniel Hack Tuke wrote of Bichat in 1872, he
found "wholly untenable the theory which would find a seat for
the emotions in any of the sympathetic ganglia." Bucke's thesis,
then, was an anachronism, a viewpoint that Alexander Bain could
only label a "peculiar conclusion."[100]

To substantiate his position Bucke relied on arguments, or, to
again quote Bain, "precarious leaps," based largely on anatomy
and analogy. The commonplace distinction between man as an
intellectual being and woman as a moral creature, he argued,
could best be explained by the observations that whereas the
average female brain was $5\frac{1}{2}$ ounces lighter than the male, her
sympathetic system, designed to serve reproductive organs lacking in men, was much larger.[101] Along a similar line, he continued, men distinguished by superior character tended to be
physically large and their sympathetic systems correspondingly
augmented. Compared to the elemental concepts of the intellect
the emotional constituents of the moral nature were much less
complicated, mirroring the relatively simple structure of the
sympathetic system when compared to the brain. Yet emotions
came from the depth of each individual, much as the sympathetic nerves, in contrast to the cerebrospinal, were buried in
the depth of the physical being. Significantly, strong emotions
were felt by the body, not the brain, a fact intuitively recog-

nized and incorporated into colloquial discourse in many languages. Finally, pathological conditions in organs with substantial sympathetic innervation, such as the adrenals in Addison's disease, inevitably resulted in "perversions of the emotional nature."[102] Though he supplemented these arguments with a variety of tortured analogies, Bucke believed anatomical inference supported the weight of his convictions.

It was essential that Bucke establish the somatic derivation of morality since upon this point rested what he regarded as his most significant contribution, a thesis doubtless confirmed during his illumination and entirely compatible with the millenarian optimism of his earlier Universalism. Man's sense of morality, he argued, had evolved in an upward fashion secondary to the evolutionary transformation of the human body in general and the sympathetic systems in specific. A comparison of "documents and works of art" of the nineteenth century with those belonging to earlier ages offered suggestive but ultimately unsatisfactory evidence of such progress. A far more convincing approach was to "adopt the development hypothesis." In so doing, it would be found that the "various inferior tribes and races of men" represented "a rough approximation" to an earlier stage in the spiritual evolution of Western man.[103] Secondly, borrowing the recapitulation theory first from Comte, and then from the German embryologist, Ernst Haeckel, he argued that the development of the individual human revealed a compressed version of the evolution of the human race. Since the child gradually evolved from relative barbarism to a mature state of moral sophistication, the human race could be assumed to follow a similar course.[104] The moral nature, then, evolved naturally with the physical evolution of the sympathetic system.

For those who accepted these observations as proof of moral evolution, Bucke offered two mechanisms by which it could be explained. The first and most significant causal factor was natural selection. Though Bain had argued that "the Moral Sentiment is about the least favourably suited for transmission by inheritance," Bucke followed Comte, who felt "the general laws of hereditary transmission" apply "to our noblest attributes as to our lowest." The latter conviction was shared by W.B. Carpenter who asserted that in man, in contrast to animals, there existed "an unlimited *capacity* for Psychical evolution" by "the genetic transmission of . . .

modification."[105] According to Bucke, characteristics conferred by a superior sympathetic nervous system equipped an individual for survival "in the struggle for existence." Fear, for example, was a facet of the moral nature that, when well developed, included a dread of death. This apprehension, in turn, prompted an individual to take precautions calculated to enhance survival and permit transmission of the trait to later generations. A highly developed moral nature also included a large capacity for love, a characteristic likely to confer a competitive advantage in seeking a mate and spawning equally moral offspring. And since an advanced moral nature was not infrequently associated with physical vigor and longevity, those who possessed it "must necessarily encroach upon the inferior individuals and races with whom they come into competition."[106] For Bucke, then, hereditary selection in large measure explained the evolution of the moral nature.

These views, however, were not rigidly deterministic, for Bucke accorded only slightly less significance to environmental influence. A child "with a certain inherited faculty of developing a more or less elevated moral nature . . . if brought up among savages . . . would acquire a moral nature . . . of a very low order." Adequate parents and home life became a means of ensuring appropriate moral development. In a similar fashion, the moral nature of great religious leaders "transmits its influence by awakening faith and love in the men and women with whom it comes in contact."[107] Unfortunately, leaders of such magnitude were uncommon, but they had their counterparts in the creative arts. Bucke followed Comte in according pride of place among artists, "the high priests of humanity," to poets. Their superior moral nature, particularly love, was conveyed through work that appealed to the emotions rather than the intellect. On exposure to poetry "a lower moral nature . . . will be improved, that is elevated," much as Bucke felt he himself had been after reading the work of Walt Whitman.[108] An inherited moral nature, then, could be nurtured by exposure to the influence of family life, religion, and art. Over time, Bucke confidently predicted, love and faith would come to dominate the moral sense, while hate and fear would persist as no more than vestigial remnants. This optimistic prediction was similar to views expressed by Comte and Carpenter, but quite at odds with those of Alexander Bain. The transcendent note on which Bucke ended his book foreshad-

owed the thesis of his later work, *Cosmic Consciousness* (1901). By
evolving toward a pure synthesis of love and faith, man's moral
nature approached a unity with the principle that animated the
universe.[109]

The response to Bucke's sweeping vision of the universal harmony inherent in the evolutionary process must have seemed to
him disproportionately diminutive. The draft manuscript was read
to Bucke's former partner, Dr. A.S. Fraser, leaving him, it appeared, speechless. No record of Harry Forman's reactions is extant, but Alfred wrote that while "greatly interesting" the book did
not lead him to change any of the views he derived from Schopenhauer. Bucke had urged a copy be sent to Benjamin Ward Richardson, insisting that "whatever he thinks of it, good or bad, that is
about What It Is Worth." Neither Richardson's response nor those
of Charles Darwin or W.B. Carpenter, to whom copies were also
sent, are known. The English mystic and socialist, Edward Carpenter, a fellow Whitmanite and friend, enjoyed the work and
ordered two extra copies.[110] Whitman himself read the volume
several times and, though ambivalent, once observed that it was "a
book you have to chew on . . . it pays principal and interest in the
end if you stick to it." It was, he continued, "worked out on daring
lines – clearly, reverently, impartially" and "scientific men are
coming around very generally to the same view."[111] This was,
indeed, a strange assessment. Far from being reverent, the medical
reviews criticized the book for "straggling indiscretions of hetero-
dox deviation from current theology" and "a suspicion of scep-
ticism."[112] Nor did these reviewers necessarily hold "the same
view," but suggested, on the contrary, that Bucke's methodology
was "fanciful."[113] Yet, significantly, though offended by his logic
and aspects of his theology, none of the reviews quarreled with the
basic assumptions upon which the book was based: The key to
understanding the human mind lay not in religion or philosophy,
but in the application of concepts such as neurological localization,
associationist psychology, and evolution. In this respect, Bucke's
neurophysiology was entirely in accord with the intellectual temper
of late-Victorian medical psychology.

Despite its idiosyncratic usages, then, *Man's Moral Nature* was a
book the genesis of which was explained by Bucke's intellectual
odyssey from Universalism to positivism, a transformation congruent with the dominant secularizing impulse in late-nineteenth

century medical thought. Many of Bucke's physician contemporaries doubtless shared in the notion that they lived at a critical juncture in history, the moment, judged by a revolution in biological thought, when man was poised on the edge of Comte's positive stage.[114] In the early nineteenth century, as Charles Rosenberg has observed, "Science and medicine, as much as Greek verbs and systematic theology, were accepted parts of a learned man's intellectual equipment."[115] But the two decades following midcentury witnessed what Robert Young has called "the fragmentation of a common context," a process in which the role of theology changed from providing a context for natural knowledge, to acting as a potential adversary of scientific learning. As theology moved toward identifying God with the unifying principles of nature, the difference between the devout and the skeptic became increasingly subtle.[116] Both Bucke and Carpenter, for example, identified a convertible form of force in the 1860s as nature's basic theme to which a Divinity became an almost extraneous afterthought. It was a small step for the diminutive but expanding Anglo-American scientific community to proclaim a distinct and formal boundary between their professional concerns and those of the theologian.[117] Though as individuals they doubtless remained committed to their traditional faiths, as a group they argued that their science was a discrete epistemological category.[118] In England and America during the 1870s physiology left behind the anatomical bias and notions of vitalism, so intimately compatible with natural theology, to pursue experimental studies, while medical psychology argued strenuously that it was a legitimate branch of biology.[119] Underlying this shift were the two key points Bucke had argued: Mind is an epiphenomenon of matter, that is, the brain, and, secondly, the body itself, is subject to precisely those natural laws operative in the inorganic world. Biomedical knowledge, in effect, assumed an esoteric character no longer accessible to an educated layperson at precisely the time at which it energetically expanded the limits of its discourse to include the new science of human behavior.

Here was a critical transformation. Health and social harmony had been closely linked from the late eighteenth century,[120] but now abstruse natural knowledge demanded mediation by medical expertise. Even a well-educated layperson could no longer aspire to the scientific understanding essential for a command of medicine's social applicability.[121] The legitimation of this new social role for medicine lay in the recondite yet objective quality of science, attributes which, as Burton Bledstein has suggested, implied "a special understanding of the universe . . . that was [it appeared] neither artificial, arbitrary, faddish, convenient, nor at the mercy of popular whim. . . ."[122] This was the secular authority that late-Victorian medicine sought and found in an increasingly technical biomedical knowledge. Indeed, as M. Jeanne Peterson perceptively concludes:

Knowledge, expertise, and science all offered an alternative system for understanding and explaining the 'real' world no longer defined in transcendental terms but in terms of the body and the material universe. The experts gained stature not because they could always act effectively, but because only they could name, describe, and explain.[123]

This, then, was the significance of Bucke's intellectual metamorphosis. The secularization of his physiology became the first step in deploying the authority of biomedical knowledge to an expanding range of social situations.

4

The social genesis of etiological speculation

In the course of formulating what he had referred to as his "speculations in moral philosophy," Bucke had familarized himself with many of the major English-language authorities on psychology and physiology. As a medical student, he had endorsed W.B. Carpenter's view that the vital principle animating human physiology is indistinguishable from the forces operative in the organic world. From his reading of Comte, Bucke learned that the laws of biology applied not only to the body, but also to the mind. Specifically, as a line of investigators from Gall to Ferrier argued, certain mental phenomena could be localized to precise sites in the nervous sytem, while their operation was often described, as in the case of Alexander Bain, in terms of associationist psychology. If mental activities were somatic in origin, they could be assumed to have evolved by the late nineteenth century, as had corporeal man, from primitive homogeneity to sophisticated complexity. This, then, was the view of mind at which Bucke had arrived by the time of his appointment to an asylum superintendency. Faced with the necessity of explaining the insanity he was expected to treat, he turned his attention from normal mental physiology to the pathology of mind. In the process his work embraced both the dominant etiological notion of late-nineteenth century somatic psychiatry—degeneration—as well as the attempt in the final decades of the century to escape the limitations of that static model by elaborating a new medical understanding of the unconscious. Though often idiosyncratic in form, his theories of psychopathology were entirely congruent with the major currents in contemporaneous psychological medicine.

By the early decades of the nineteenth century, lunacy had clearly been designated a medical disorder and most physicians would have endorsed the assertion that mind was a function of brain.[1] The "Mind and the Brain," proclaimed W.B. Carpenter's study of mental physiology, "not withstanding those differences in properties which place them in different philosophical categories, are . . . intimately blended in their *actions.*" His views were often relied upon by Daniel H. Tuke and J.C. Bucknill in *A Manual of Psychological Medicine,* the most popular English-language work for students and practitioners from its appearance in 1858 to its fourth edition in 1879. The authors had no hesitation in concluding: "*the existence of any pathological state in the organ of mind will interrupt the function of that organ, and produce a greater or less amount of disease of mind – that is, insanity.*" Though their book was displaced in popularity by Henry Maudsley's *Pathology of Mind* (1879), their somatic view of insanity was firmly endorsed in the newer work.[2] The behavioral aberrations of the insane mind were, physicians agreed, simply the symptoms of a diseased brain.

If there was a medical consensus as to the somatic source of lunacy, there was also substantial agreement among alienists on the manner in which the cerebral pathology originated and the specific nature of the lesions involved. In the first half of the century, though purely physical agents were occasionally assigned a causal role, "moral" or psychological events were given clear prominence. Loss or grief, disappointment in love or business, religious or political excitement, inadequate rearing or schooling, all might be found to account for more cases of insanity than either physical causes such as intoxication, sexual excess and blows to the head, or hereditary influences.[3] Such causes, however, were not to be considered entirely psychological rather than somatic, for they did, indeed, cause changes in the brain. Bucknill and Tuke admitted that microscopic alterations were often not present in the brains of deceased lunatics, a fact that they believed justified their functional view of organic pathology. Certainly, it was an argument sufficiently persuasive to receive support from many of their contemporaries, including John P. Gray, the venerable editor of the *American Journal of Insanity.*[4] Just as strong emotions might cause the dilation of facial vessels to produce a blush, so strong psychological forces might result in vascular congestion of the brain. With the ensuing stagnation of blood flow, the brain would be deprived of

nutrition while toxic waste would accumulate. Vascular congestion was, in turn, a hallmark of inflammation, a process that, in
the brain, caused an initial area of local irritation that quickly
became generalized. It was this irritable brain which produced
the excited behavior or, after prolonged stimulation, the lethargy, that defined the spectrum of insanity.[5] Though aware that
some might quarrel with "the congestion theory of the pathology of insanity," Tuke and Bucknill considered it far superior to
"the fantastic alliance of spurious physiology and Kantian metaphysics" of those who denied the cellular basis of cerebral
pathology.[6] Though the causes of insanity, then, might be psychological, the resulting pathology was wholly somatic.[7]

In the second half of the nineteenth century, alienists began to
change the emphasis in their etiological theory. No new concepts
were introduced, but a qualification was appended to the previous credo: In order for psychological forces to induce insanity, a
hereditary predisposition was often necessary.[8] When John
Conolly wrote on insanity in the 1830s, he conceded that certain
character types in the tradition of humoral theory seemed predisposed to particular mental aberrations. His contemporary,
George Man Burrows, assigned an even greater significance to
familial traits as a predisposing etiological factor.[9] But neither
suggested a diathesis with the dogmatic enthusiasm later expressed by Henry Maudsley. "The germs of insanity are most
often latent in the character," the latter wrote, "and the final
outbreak is the explosion of a long train of antecedent preparations."[10] How many patients had inherited "what might be
called the insane temperament" remained uncertain, but Maudsley, like Isaac Ray before him, estimated as many as half of all
cases and expected future research to reveal a higher proportion.[11] Certainly, some alienists continued to stress the primacy
of environmental causation, particularly, as in the case of George
M. Beard, the tensions associated with modern civilization.[12] But
in the final two decades of the nineteenth century the emphasis
on heredity appeared to transcend its cautious status as a mere
diathesis, to become the single most significant etiological factor
in accounting for madness.[13] The "most important predisposing
cause of insanity," wrote the neurologist, Edward Spitzka, "is
undoubtedly . . . hereditary transmission of structural and physiological defects of the central nervous apparatus."[14] It was a

judgment that many were to echo[15] and some, Bucke among them, to expand.

Bucke's speculations on mental pathology were based on his often-repeated belief that man's mind had evolved from

the imperfect sensation of the worm, the rudimentary sight, hearing, and taste of the fish and reptile; and the simple consciousness which, springing from these, passed to us after almost infinite ages of slow evolution and amelioration through tens of thousands of generations of placental mammals our immediate progenitors.[16]

That this position provoked a skeptical response among some physicians doubtless came as a surprise to Bucke, for he emphasized that his authorities were the leading figures in British biology. Francis Galton, for example, wrote "a good size volume to prove that genius is hereditary,"[17] while "the general theory of psychic evolution" was "propounded by the best writers on the subject such as Darwin and Romanes."[18] Taking his initial cue from Charles Lyell's belief that language paralleled the evolution of the species, Bucke scoured works by philologists for evidence of man's intellectual progress.[19] Without speech in which to embody concepts, wrote the linguistic theorist, Max Müller, reason was impossible.[20] But speech itself had been shown to have grown slowly "by natural selection and the struggle for existence."[21] To Bucke the implication was clear: The intellect, as he had earlier argued of the moral nature, had clearly evolved in the recent past. Such philological arguments were a popular form of evidence, finding a place in Robert Chambers' *Vestiges of the Natural History of Creation* (1844)[22] and forming the principal scaffold upon which George Romanes based his *Mental Evolution in Man* (1888).[23] Indeed, Müller himself had argued that linguistics was "one of the physical sciences," and yet unique in that it allowed scholars to establish "a frontier between man and the beast" at a time when other sciences pointed in precisely the opposite direction.[24] Deploying philological speculations, then, was to Bucke and his contemporaries an entirely legitimate method of investigating the archeology of the mind.

At this point in his theory of insanity, Bucke introduced what he called the *pivot fact:* though both the cognitive and affective portions of mind had evolved together, not all aspects of the mind were of the same age. In support of this contention, he marshaled two arguments, both drawn from current biology. First, he asserted, "the evolution of the individual is necessarily a repetition in a condensed form of the evolution of the race."[25] Bucke may have first encountered this argument while reading works by Comte or Spencer,[26] though the idea was by no means new to the nineteenth century.[27] The major spokesman for the belief that "ontogeny is nothing else but phylogeny"[28] was Ernst Haeckel, Darwin's champion in Germany. This theory he designated the *biogenetic law*, and believed it held the promise, through embryological studies, of tracing the path of human evolution.[29] This, certainly, was the purpose to which Bucke put the concept. He argued that the newborn child lacked a moral sense in exactly the same fashion as had primitive man during the childlike phase of human evolution. It was a view of the recent derivation and fragility of the moral nature that the eminent English alienist, Henry Maudsley, shared.[30] Such reasoning was primarily useful in conjunction with a second piece of evidence. According to Darwin's work on the breeding of animals, the most recently acquired characteristics were the most subject to lapse.[31] Among humans, for example, it appeared that one in sixty individuals lacked color sense. That this was a recently acquired faculty Bucke believed was established by the work of the philologist, Lazarus Geiger, who claimed that from the absence of words signifying colours in ancient language, one could infer an inability to discriminate color.[32] If, then, newly evolved characteristics were most subject to lapse, and since, as recapitulation theory and linguistic evidence suggested, the moral nature and the intellect were recently acquired attributes, man's mind was at high risk for developmental failure.[33]

Bucke was now prepared to state his "main thesis – that insanity is essentially the breaking down of mental faculties which are unstable chiefly because they are recent."[34] The insane were "nothing more or less than cases of atavism" who illustrated "reversion to an ancestral type."[35] In these unfortunate individuals, the normal bonds of association between simple concepts and primary emotional states, which had slowly evolved in the race, dissolved and were replaced by others that were "trivial, valueless, mischievous."[36] Insanity was, then, simply regression to an earlier and primitive state of being. It was a view Bucke found in his reading of works by Prosper Despine, Havelock Ellis, Enrico

Ferri, Cesare Lombroso, Richard von Krafft-Ebing, and many other European physicians or social theorists.[37] Like these individuals, Bucke believed that, "The great matter is heredity . . . everything is transmitted – physical traits – moral traits." Against a degenerative taint, environmental manipulation was powerless.[38] Indeed, the environment was relevant only in explaining the first appearance of degeneracy in a given family, alcoholism being a favored example.[39] All alienists, Bucke concluded, would accept the validity of this atavistic theory, unless "there is some extraordinary individual who has not taken up the entire theory of evolution as a reading man and a scientist."[40]

Bucke may well have been correct in his belief that the majority of his medical contemporaries accepted the broad outlines of his view of insanity. The influence of the recapitulation hypothesis, Stephen Jay Gould has suggested, "as an import from evolutionary theory into other fields was exceeded only by natural selection itself," while its principal spokesman, Ernst Haeckel, has been described as "the most colorful and the most puzzling natural scientist on the European Continent during the heady rise of evolutionary theory."[41] Nor was the communication of the theory·restricted to an academic audience. Haeckel's major popular work, *The Riddle of the Universe* (1899), sold 100,000 copies in its first year, passed through ten editions by 1919, and was translated into twenty-five languages.[42] References to recapitulation appeared in nonscientific sources, such as the poetry of Rudyard Kipling or Alfred Tennyson,[43] and a number of notable Victorian medical and social theorists accorded it an important role in their thought. Sigmund Freud, for example, a convinced Lamarckian, observed that each "individual somehow recapitulates in an abbreviated form the entire development of the race."[44] Repression could be interpreted as an attempt to mask the primal urges of previous, less-evolved generations, while the oral-anal aspect of infantile sexuality recalled an earlier quadrupedal ancestry governed by smell and taste.[45] Similarly, George Stanley Hall, the founder of American child psychology, based his views of childhood development and appropriate educational methods on Haeckel's theories. His ideas were to spill over into countless local school boards in the United States, where the curricula were formulated so as to guide pupils in their journey from primal savagery to civilized maturity.[46] Among other scholars who adopted recapitulation were Edward D. Cope, the leading paleontologist and comparative anatomist in late nineteenth-century America; J. W. Draper, the popular intellectual historian of Europe; Carl Jung, Freud's associate; and Benjamin Kidd, the celebrated English Social Darwinist.[47]

Why did recapitulation strike such a responsive cord? In part, the theory owed its appeal to its inherent flexibility. To the social optimist it appeared to confirm a faith in mankind's progressive ascent from primitive barbarism, while conversely, to a conservative, it documented the thinly veiled savagery of human nature. Undoubtedly its most important appeal, however, lay in its biological determinism. Replete with statistics, graphs, and embryological diagrams, Haeckel's work spoke with the authoritative vocabulary of the laboratory. It was a mode of discourse that testified to the value-transcendent character of the scientific knowledge it conveyed. And this objective knowledge, in turn, promised a positive embryological answer to the question of man's ancestry with which neither incomplete fossil remains nor archeological evidence could compete. It allowed, in fact, the construction of a fundamental equation: Primitive man was like the modern child. This was a useful simile for, once established, any behavior judged as childlike against the norm of the Western European adult invited comparison with primitive forebears or simian antecedents. At particular risk as subjects for such comparisons were the insane and the criminal. Indeed, as the works of criminologists revealed,[48] the doctrine of recapitulation found a critical corollary in the theory of atavism.

Signifying regression to a more primitive evolutionary state, atavism was a refinement of the somewhat older and more general concept of degeneration, associated with mid-century French psychiatry. Jacques Moreau de Tours suggested the pivotal message of this group in the 1850s when he argued that heredity was "the source of nine-tenths of mental disease."[49] In a two-volume work published between 1847 and 1850, Prosper Lucas also emphasized the role of heredity in the etiology of nervous disorders and suggested that such inherited diseases could change form to display different symptomatology in subsequent generations.[50] The latter concept, designated polymorphic inheritance, together with a firm belief in the Lamarckian transmission of acquired characteristics were central to the thought of the most widely known of the early degeneration theorists, Benedict Morel. While he was willing to concede an important pathogenic role to environmental factors such as intoxicants, inheritance assumed the central role in his explanation for the cause of both insanity and criminality. He introduced the *law of progressivity,* which employed polymorphic inheritance to argue that an afflicted family might begin as simply nervous only to degenerate via psychosis and idiocy to sterility by the fourth generation. Such mental deviants, he felt, could also be identified by morphological stigmata such as pointed ears, stunted growth or cranial abnormalities.[51] Morel's work incorporated a religious perspective and explicitly rejected the theory of evolution. Both of these characteristics were absent from the work of his best-known successor, the neuropathologist, Valentin Magnan. He based his view of degeneration on the hypothesis that the process had its origin in an inherited "special brain structure" in the predisposed individual.[52] Couched in the language of neuroanatomy so popular with a generation impressed by the results of cerebral localization, his studies became standard references on the subject. They were complemented by similar assumptions in Richard von Krafft-Ebing's work on sexual pathology, J.-M. Charcot's on hysteria, and the neuropathological studies of Moriz Benedikt.[53]

In the final decades of the nineteenth century, the doctrine of degeneration spread beyond medicine to become a topic of popular concern. Max Nordau, for example, discussed literary and cultural decline in a hotly debated volume that appeared in English in 1895. Earlier, in 1877, Richard Dugdale had created a sensation in the United States with his study of the malignant descent of the debauched Jukes family over the course of more than 100 years.[54] But undoubtedly the area in which degeneration theory enjoyed its greatest popularity was in a new field closely allied to psychiatry, that of criminology. Its acknowledged founder was, in fact, an Italian physician, Cesare Lombroso, whose work encompassed the as–yet undifferentiated fields of forensic psychiatry, comparative anatomy, and anthropology. The Italian School had its opponents, particularly the environmentalist studies of Gabriel Tarde, but until the appearance of Charles Goring's *The English Convict* in 1913 and William

Healy's *The Individual Delinquent* the following year, Lombroso's ideas on "criminal man" dominated criminological theory.[55] Like many physicians of his day, Bucke included, Lombroso fell under the influence of Comte. Following the lead of the phrenologist, Franz Joseph Gall, he attempted to develop a science of physical deformities by which to identify the mentally abnormal. He was familiar with Morel's theory of degeneration to which he gave a new Darwinian twist by arguing that such regression was, in fact, a reversion to an earlier ancestral type. By way of proof, again like Bucke, he used the recapitulation theory to equate criminality with a stage in normal childhood, in turn a reflection of savage progenitors. Physical stigmata and deviant behavior together defined atavism which, when transmitted to later generations, resulted in degeneration.[56] It was a concept that reached English-speaking audiences well before the ideas delineated in his *L'Uomo Delinquente* (1876) were made available in an abridged translation in 1911. Havelock Ellis, for example, reviewed European criminal anthropology in *The Criminal,* published in 1890, as did a number of other authors in scholarly journals.[57] In testimony to the success of these reviews in conveying degeneration theory, during the final decade of the century, several studies of criminals appeared in America that adopted Lombroso's approach to hereditary degeneration.[58] Though the concept was to lose its luster in criminology by the First World War, it influenced, to varying degrees, the eugenics movement,[59] imperial theorists,[60] and psychiatry.

Psychiatry, in fact, was often indistinguishable from criminology, its practitioners claiming expertise on deviant behavior in both fields.[61] Lombroso himself, of course, had been a physician at several asylums, and he readily conceded his indebtedness to British alienists, ranging from James Pritchard to Henry Maudsley.[62] Indeed, of degenerates the latter wrote, "Crime is a sort of outlet in which their unsound tendencies are discharged; they would go mad if they were not criminals."[63] Maudsley became the principal English-speaking authority on psychopathology in the late nineteenth century, following the publication of his *Physiology and Pathology of Mind* (1867) and *Responsibility in Mental Disease* (1874).[64] Like Bucke, Maudsley had early fallen under the spell of Comte, had endorsed W.B. Carpenter's physiochemical interpretation of vital force, and was given to utopian views of human evolution.[65] He read and appreciated Morel's work on degeneration, coming to share his view that "Insanity . . . may be looked upon . . . as a stage in the descent toward sterile idiocy." This "retrograde movement" of a degenerate group of humans was, he felt, likely due to a functional "intrinsic disorder of nerve element itself,"[66] which time might establish as essentially chemical in nature.[67]

Many Anglo-American physicians adopted Maudsley's views in their own publications, often, as in the case of Eugene Talbot, losing sight of his frequent caveats, to create a rigid determinism.[68] Indeed, even the most innovative neuropsychiatric theorists of the day incorporated elements of degeneration theory. Insanity, argued Hughlings Jackson, was a dissolution of the higher nervous centers, allowing the disinhibition of more primitive neurological functions. It was a sophisticated neurophysiological view of etiology that in some respects resembled the earlier views of the degeneration theorist, Magnan.[69] In the United States, Adolf Meyer, the energetic neuropathologist associated with the early mental hygiene movement, was critical of degeneration theory in 1896. But his criticism was directed at the lack of scientific rigor in the work of degeneration theorists rather than at any flaw in their hypothesis itself. Indeed, he set himself the task of explaining to his less-enlightened alienist colleagues the most efficacious means of measuring "morphological deviations from the normal" in asylum patients, so as to verify statistically the physical stigmata of degeneracy.[70] Hereditary degeneration, then, with varying degrees of determinism, became a central organizing concept of late nineteenth-century psychiatry.

Bucke was familiar with the work on degeneration by authorities such as Lombroso and Maudsley. That he was receptive to their arguments may in part by explained by his earlier exposure to the idea in Comte's philosophy,[71] and by the fact that eminent physicians such as Rudolf Virchow devoted considerable discussion to the mechanism of atavism.[72] Even Darwin himself lent his scientific stature to a cautious endorsement of Maudsley's view of degeneration.[73] But beyond the scientific imprimatur conveyed by the collective work of these scholarly authorities, Bucke and other late-nineteenth century alienists had pragmatic professional motives for enthusiastically endorsing degeneration as an etiological reality. Based on the theory of physical evolution, it substantiated the somatic model of mental illness necessary for the legitimation of the alienists' claims to expertise. Postmortem examination had consistently failed to document gross or microscopic lesions in the brains of the insane, an embarrassment that forced physicians to posit functional rather than structural lesions. The existence of a hereditary neuropathic diathesis, suddenly made overt by situational stress or vice, provided an important explanation for the manner in which these functional deficits operated: They were, in Maudsley's phrase, "intranervine so to speak."[74] Since the majority of the asylum's long-term patients were assumed to suffer from such inherited neurological taints, few cures were to be expected. Degeneration theory appeared to exempt alienists from any responsibility for the depressing decline in cure rates in late nineteenth-century asylums.[75] It also removed from criticism the often austere and crowded facilities that governments provided for the insane. Even the alienists themselves were forced to accept the adequacy of custodial institutions since, for the incurable, the pleasant environment earlier advocated by proponents of moral therapy was a luxury rather than a therapeutic necessity. Finally, if physicians were absolved from criticism of their inability to cure, they, in turn, gained a powerful weapon with which to assault their detractors. The incidence of mental illness was widely believed to be increasing in the late nineteenth century.[76] Since it was in substantial measure the result of a hereditary taint, its control became primarily a social, rather than strictly medical, problem. The locus of responsibility shifted to the courts, legislatures, schools, and churches, but with the important caveat that the physician would provide expert direction on matters ranging from mental competence in law to the principles of eugenics. Degeneration theory, in effect, lifted alienists from the stigma of therapeutic defeat to the pedestal of social prophecy.

Degeneration, then, gratified specific professional needs for late-nineteenth century psychiatry. But it also served a larger and more covert social role. Consider the popular work on insanity published in 1878 by Dr. Daniel Hack Tuke. The concerned layperson or practitioner would learn that paupers, individuals from a "stratum of civilized society which is squalid, and drunken and sensual," were disproportionately represented in asylums. A simple "South Sea Islander," though savage, would be less likely to "transgress the laws of mental health" than would a "Wiltshire labourer." Because of dissolute habits, or "the brain he inherited from parents indulging in like habits," the English laborer was "more liable to insanity than other people." The initial impetus for debauched behavior that began the degeneration process, Tuke believed, was inherent in the political and economic organization of European civilization. "The atmosphere which the Englishman and the Frenchman breathe," he wrote, "is full of psychological germs calculated to infect the nervous system with disease." The result visited upon the poor was actually "worse than the condition of savages" in its social implications. The savage had not yet evolved; the lunatic poor fell back and beyond this primitive but pure state, as a consequence of vice. "Recklessness, drunkenness, poverty, misery characterize the class," he concluded, "no wonder that from such a source spring the hopelessly incurable lunatics who crowd pauper asylums, to the horror of ratepayers." There was no mistaking Tuke's message: poverty, degeneration, and lunacy were all cut of the same cloth.[77]

The hereditary determinism underlying views such as those expressed by Tuke have been characterized as a secular philosophy designed to replace religious conviction as a means of imposing structure on the spectacle of a disorderly Victorian world. Not only did it explain, but it promised, by society's adherence to the laws of inheritance, stability and continuity of social norms.[78] Beyond this reassuring vision, however, lay a fundamental statement about social relationships in the nineteenth century. Even a cursory acquaintance with public mental institutions confirmed Tuke's belief that their inhabitants were largely drawn from the ranks of the poor. It was psychiatry that introduced the crucial concept that the insane were also degenerates, nature's castoffs hurtling down the evolutionary staircase. It was now possible to forge a basic equation; poverty and degeneracy, in the asylum, were clearly synonymous. Little imagination was required to hypothesize that what applied within the mental institution was equally applicable to other dependent social categories, such as criminals, and, ultimately, to the poor as a class. Rather than viewing the poverty-stricken as casualties of an inequitable industrial capitalism, physicians and social theorists labeled them atavistic misfits in an otherwise evolving world. It was not simply the appearance of Darwin's work in the 1850s that explained the drift toward biological reductionism for, as Charles Rosenberg has argued, the content of scientific views of heredity changed little over the course of the century.[79] Rather, it was in these years that the urban poor became permanently, relentlessly visible, a phenomenon for which hereditarian thought appeared to provide a ready scientific explanation.

The work of theorists such as Morel, Moreau, and their successors was shaped by exactly this social reality.[80] The presence of poverty was not, of course, new to mid-nineteenth century Europe; the poor had increased rapidly in the final years of the eighteenth century and provided a not-infrequent focus of social debate.[81] But what did change noticeably at midcentury was the moral and biological significance attached to destitution. In Paris the industrial proletariat was equated with savagery and identified by the hereditary physical stigmata of ugliness, deformity, and disease. Crime, formerly tinged in middle-class literature with an exotic quality, became simply the prosaic province of the urban poor. Once morally neutral, the Parisian indigents had become the "dangerous classes" by 1850.[82] Nor was this perceptual transformation confined to the Continent. Local English statistical societies had, since the 1830s, shown a dynamic interest in the collection of "moral statistics," the analysis of which suggested that the poor were often both heathen and criminal.[83] But it was the evocative and detailed portrait of London poverty sketched by Henry Mayhew in the pages of the *Morning Chronicle* late in 1849 that "seized public interest in a way which has scarcely ever been equalled in British journalism."[84] Several factors combined to spur this middle-class curiosity. In the wake of the Poor Law Amendment Act of 1834, the percentage of the population eligible for relief fell quickly, casting a significant number of paupers into new roles, whether as vagrants, recipients of tenuous private charity, or the lowest category of working poor.[85] Legislation, in effect, had made poverty more visible, and it was made even more so by the ensuing Chartist agitation, punctuated by devastating epidemics of cholera.

While Mayhew's descriptive acuity remained uncommon, his approach was widely emulated in provincial cities and a steady trickle of urban exposés appeared during the 1860s. Implicit in these revelations was a warning of the physical and spiritual danger posed by poverty in general and a newly discovered sub-species, the lowest stratum of the poor, the "dangerous class," in particular.[86] Social disorders in London in the late 1860s were seen as vivid proof of the demoralization of the poor, a view confirmed by the more-extensive disruptions two decades later. By the 1880s poverty, again a topic of journalistic interest, was perceived by the English middle class with fear more than compassion. Both the existence of the social residuum, the submerged tenth of destitute and depraved, and the presumed cause, hereditary degeneration, had become familiar concepts to the Victorians. The investigations of Charles Booth and Benjamin Rowntree, meliorist in intent, simply served to document statistically the pervasive dimensions of poverty's threat.[87] In effect, after 1850 poverty in Britain and France was perceived in increasingly hereditarian terms and, equally, conferred the stigma of moral incapacity on its victims. The degeneration theory proposed by mid-nineteenth-century French psychiatry, then, was both a product of these middle-class fears and, as the century progressed, an increasingly important source of scientific legitimation for the theory's basic assumptions.

Though initially a product of Old World class divisions, degeneration theory was welcomed in North America as well, for here, too, poverty was "discovered" in the mid-nineteenth century. In fact, poverty in the new world was even more sinister, for it either challenged the comfortable myth of America's social uniqueness[88] or it suggested that those who failed to attain affluence in a land of inherent opportunity were individuals devoid of industry or ability. It was during the 1840s, a period of frequent social disorder in the wake of massive immigration, financial panics, and urban growth, that middle-class Americans recognized the prevalence of poverty. If compassion was one response, the rhetoric frequently used to describe the poor – debased, vicious, abandoned – suggested that revulsion was an even more pervasive reaction.[89] Likewise in Canada, the poor were both conspicuous and unwelcome. The harsh winters were found not to be the socially invigorating and purifying process celebrated by poets, but an annual period of hardship for the nation's poor.[90] As in the United States, many of this class had arrived as penniless immigrants in the 1830s and quickly became a permanent feature of the social landscape.[91] In fact, as early as 1837, the

focus of public relief shifted from recent arrivals to the indige-
nous poor, with one-twelfth of Toronto's population in receipt
of aid from the newly opened House of Industry.[92] In both
Canada[93] and the United States the purveyors of charity were
obsessed with the distinction between the deserving poor – those
who through age, illness, or misfortune fell victim to poverty –
and the undeserving, the depraved whose improvident and in-
temperate character was justly rewarded by indigence. As the
visibility of the poor increased, so too did the conviction that
poverty was intimately linked to crime[94] and that both of these
characteristics, once established, became hereditary.[95] In North
America, as in Europe, poverty and moral degeneracy had become a truism of social theory by the end of the century.

Such is not to suggest that the medical proponents of degeneration theory were intent upon grinding the faces of the poor.
On the contrary, Lombroso, for example, like Bucke, considered
himself a socialist, and his young colleague, Enrico Ferri, was an
ardent Marxist.[96] Many of the late nineteenth-century physicians
and anthropologists who studied the inheritance of lunacy or
criminality correctly viewed themselves as leaders of the liberal
intelligentsia.[97] Armed with empirical evidence as to the cause
and management of deviance, these positivists were convinced
that both society and its misfits would ultimately benefit from
alterations in social policy. Yet beyond this level of individual
motivation these theorists were confined in their analyses by the
parameters of the class divisions within which they themselves
existed. The ultimate effect of their degeneration message was to
naturalize social forms, to legitimate, in the value-transcendent
language of science, existing class relationships.[98] If poverty was
a product of a biological process, it was decreed by a natural
order unresponsive to human intervention. Degeneration theory
was, in part, the product of nineteenth-century class divisions
and at once a significant argument by which these divisions could
be justified and perpetuated.

The psychiatric fascination with degenerates did not disappear
by the end of the nineteenth century; on the contrary, it was
asserted with a vengeance just before the First World War in the
campaign against the "threat" of the feebleminded.[99] But the fact
remained that the pool of degenerates – that is the very poor – was
steadily receding into invisiblity. Partially through the growth of

welfare institutions such as the asylum itself, the desperate poor were, if not reduced in number, sequestered from view. In effect, by its very success in corraling the degenerate, psychiatry was in danger of losing the social rationale behind its theories. It was clearly time to seek a new clientele, to move beyond the narrow confines of the asylum and its degenerate inhabitants. The transformation, neither abrupt nor rapid, was clearly evident after the First World War when it was expressed most dramatically in the mental hygiene movement. This earnest group sought out otherwise-normal individuals who, under stress, might become emotionally disturbed. Admittedly the older hereditarian orientation lingered in popular thought, for a contemporary of the mental hygiene campaign was the dynamic eugenics movement dedicated to the suppression of inferior human stock.[100] But psychiatry now chose to go its own way. It would establish that even within the ostensibly sound cerebrums of the growing middle class, untainted by hereditary blight, lurked the unconscious potential for mental aberration. The discovery of the unconscious, in short, was to provide psychiatry with both a new clientele and a vastly enhanced social authority.

With the publication in 1901 of his final book, *Cosmic Consciousness* (Figure 11), Bucke joined the groping but relentless search for a new medical understanding of the unconscious mind. He viewed the work as part of a trilogy. In *Man's Moral Nature* he had sketched his optimistic, evolutionary view of the human mind and predicted continued spiritual growth. His biographical study, *Walt Whitman,* appeared four years later and argued that the "Good Grey Poet" was an individual example of a new stage in moral elevation. In his final work, he assigned to that elevation the term cosmic consciousness and explained the mechanism by which it would, eventually, be shared by all men. It was clearly a message that appealed to twentieth-century readers for over the next eight decades an additional eight publishers brought out editions of the book, some of these reprinted many times, and a German translation appeared in 1975.[101] Among Bucke's contemporaries, however, his ideas met a mixed reception. None of the major Anglo-American journals of neurology or psychiatry accorded his book a review. His friend, William Osler, sent a note of congratulations and William James, the Harvard psychologist, reprinted a passage in his classic study of

COSMIC CONSCIOUSNESS: A STUDY
IN THE EVOLUTION OF THE HUMAN
MIND, EDITED BY DR. RICHARD
MAURICE BUCKE

*Verily, verily I say unto thee, except a man be born anew he cannot see the
kingdom of God.*

INNES & SONS
100 SOUTH TENTH STREET
PHILADELPHIA
1901

Figure 11. Title page from *Cosmic Consciousness* (1901). Source: R. M.
Bucke, *Cosmic Consciousness* (Philadelphia: Innes and Sons, 1901).

religious experience. When he first explained the notion of cosmic
consciousness to his close friend Harry Forman, or a former
McGill classmate, John Harkness, he was met with polite skepticism. [102] But to Bucke himself the volume held immense significance. On a conscious level it allowed him to pay tribute to the
most important relationship of his adult life, his friendship with
Walt Whitman; in a more covert sense, it provided an opportunity
to focus his cherished biological perspective on an otherwise metaphysical topic. In the final analysis, the book, an eclectic blend of
hero worship, exotic religion, and science, assumes significance
not as a classic of mysticism but as a specific example of psychological medicine's attempt at the end of the nineteenth century to
extend its domain to previously private and hidden functions of
the subconscious mind. If, to later generations, Bucke's study of

what he called cosmic consciousness has a curious mystical tone, to at least some of his contemporaries it must have seemed as plausible as the early work of Freud or Janet.

Though the book shared the major themes found in his two earlier works, his fascination with the specific notion of cosmic consciousness seemed to date from November of 1891. It was then that he wrote to Walt Whitman's constant companion, Horace Traubel, that he had begun putting his ideas on paper. Four months later he predicted a rather large book with Whitman as the "central figure . . . but the bulk of the space . . . taken up by other men and by exhibition and explanation." He urged Traubel, Whitman, and another of the poet's admirers, John H. Johnston, to share with him details of any experiences that resembled his own illumination in 1872, an event that had become in Bucke's mind the prototype for the receipt of cosmic consciousness. As well, from the English mystic, Edward Carpenter, he solicited advice on the "Theosophic theory of the Cosmic Sense."[103] The results of his inquiries first saw print in 1893 as an essay entitled "Walt Whitman and the Cosmic Sense." A more theoretical paper, "Cosmic Consciousness," was presented to the annual meeting of the American Medico–Psychological Association in 1894. Portions of this essay formed the conclusion of his 1897 presidential address to the Psychological Section of the British Medical Association under the title, "Mental Evolution in Man."[104] Though he predicted to Harry Forman that he would be "held up by the smart journals as a first class ignoramus," his thoughts assumed book form by 1901. Satisfied with the finished product – "the handsomest book I have ever seen" – he confided to a friend, "I have shown that there really is a world beyond this realm of self-consciousness infinitely more important than the old one we used to think we knew."[105] Sadly, his accidental death in 1902 prevented him from savoring the popularity his work was to enjoy.

Much of the introduction to *Cosmic Consciousness* would have been familiar to those acquainted with Bucke's earlier work. Once again he argued that the human mind, both the moral spirit and the intellect, had evolved, and based his case on examples of linguistic development and the gradual acquisition of color sense. Not all human capacities, he cautioned, developed at a similar rate, as the recapitulation theory suggested. Just as each individual moved from embryonic form, through birth, to adult consciousness, so the human race had sequentially acquired discrete characteristics which moved it from barbarism to its sophisticated nineteenth-century level of mental development. It was the latter process that was the point of departure for what was new in the book. Citing the theories of George Romanes, the British zoologist–psychologist, he asserted that humans initially shared with the advanced animal world *simple consciousness,* an awareness of both the environment and the somatic self. Over countless eons, largely through mechanisms explained by associationist psychology, man evolved *self consciousness.* By virtue of this faculty, humans were able to perceive themselves as distinct entities apart from the rest of the universe and to engage in the process of deliberate introspection. It was a giant step from primitive animality, but it was dwarfed by the magnitude of what Bucke believed was to come: Mankind was on the threshold of a new level of awareness, best labeled cosmic consciousness.[106]

The new faculty was by no means easily defined. Bucke himself had dimly glimpsed its potential during his illumination in 1872, but only after years of contemplation understood its true meaning.[107] In essence, it signified a profound understanding "of the life and order of the universe."[108] More specifically, wrote Bucke,

This consciousness shows the cosmos to consist not of dead matter governed by unconscious, rigid, and unintending law; it shows it on the contrary as entirely immaterial, entirely spiritual and entirely alive; it shows that death is an absurdity, that every one and everything has eternal life; it shows that the universe is God and that God is the universe, and that no evil ever did or ever will enter into it.[109]

At least fifty men in world history were known to have had such insight, including Jesus, Mohammed, Buddha, Paul, Dante, Bacon, Bucke himself, and, towering above all others, Walt Whitman. After reviewing his fourteen certain and thirty-six possible cases of cosmic consciousness, Bucke arrived at a significant conclusion: The incidence of cosmic insight was increasing and would "become more and more universal and appear earlier in the individual life until the race at large will possess this faculty."[110] Here, then, was the essential thesis of *Cosmic Conscious-*

ness. A new but natural power latent in the contemporaneous mind was to fundamentally alter the course of human history.

How is one to account for this millenarian view of a new form of consciousness, seemingly at odds with the materialism of Bucke's medical philosophy? Bucke, himself, believed his cosmic theory simply derived from years of empirical study of Walt Whitman's character and his principal work, *Leaves of Grass*.[111] This assumption remains unchallenged in the work of most scholars who have encountered Bucke in the course of investigating Whitman's career. He appears in the pages of Gay Wilson Allen's study largely as a sycophant who naively assigned to Whitman "the character of a saint." More recently, Justin Kaplan has written that "Bucke's devotion was so intense and of such long standing that over the years he came to look like Whitman. Sometimes he even fancied he was Whitman . . . ."[112] Yet a close examination of Bucke's relationship with the poet fails to document a significant influence on the evolution of his thought. Rather, it is clear that Bucke, in the early 1870s, read into Whitman's poetry ideas with which he was already familiar, and that, in later years, he personified in the poet values he himself admired. Whitman realized this when he explained to a friend that Bucke, when they first met, was already "given to Oriental studies" and simply assumed "the things he had been dreaming about" were embodied in the poems of his new friend.[113] In fact, over time Bucke may well have come to influence Whitman's own perception of his poetry. After reading Bucke's biography of him Whitman confessed to Edward Carpenter, "I thought there was a germinal idea in Bucke's book – the idea that 'Leaves of Grass' was above all an expression of the Moral Nature."[114] But in neither their infrequent personal encounters nor in their remarkably pedestrian correspondence[115] did they discuss at any length philosophical or literary concepts. To Whitman, Bucke became primarily an empathetic source of medical attention and he confided to a friend that it was only in a medical context that one could "thoroughly know, comprehend" Bucke.[116] (Figure 12.) For his part, during the 1880s, Bucke found that it was his friend's illness rather than his ideas that demanded his constant attention.

If the ideas in *Cosmic Consciousness* drew little from Bucke's relationship with Whitman, they did share similarities with con-

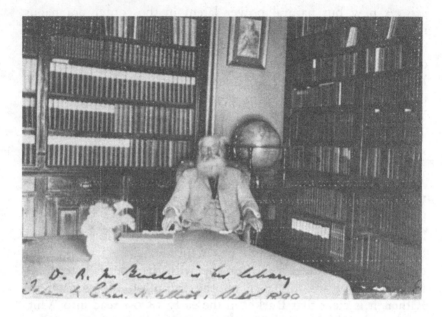

Figure 12. R. M. Bucke in his library at the London Asylum, 1899. A portrait of Walt Whitman is visible in the background. Source: R. M. Bucke Collection, University of Western Ontario.

cepts Bucke had encountered in his youth. Universalist theology, for example, predicted ultimate salvation for all men and defined that redemption in dangerously secular terms as essentially a union with the universal divine spirit. The physiology of W.B. Carpenter established that all bodily systems were subject to the laws prevalent elsewhere in creation, a thesis that allowed Bucke to apply the optimistic evolutionary doctrine to the human mind. Finally, in the work of Comte, Bucke encountered the religion of humanity, in which mankind itself was deified when it attained the positivist stage, as the ultimate achievement of the universe. That Bucke chose to express these eclectic personal influences in the visionary form of *Cosmic Consciousness* was consistent, as well, with both a tradition of utopian medical literature dating to classical antiquity, and with a flurry of such writing among Victorian authors. His friend, Benjamin Ward Richardson, spoke to physicians and laymen in his popular description of an urban utopia entitled "Hygeia: A City of Health." Similarly, Havelock Ellis published a Bellamy-style assessment of nineteenth-century society from the vantage point of a future utopia in which medicine, among other things, had vastly improved.[117] But neither personal beliefs nor the popularity of late nineteenth-century futuristic literature alone account for the shape and substance of Bucke's book. Rather, to a significant degree, the explanation for the book's genesis lies in the turbulent world of fin-de-siècle medical psychology.

During the 1880s when Bucke's ideas on cosmic consciousness were nascent, the validity of the prevailing somatic paradigm in psychiatry was under attack by radical formulations the origins of which stretched back to the 1850s. It was in that decade that a wave of spiritualism, a belief that affirmed the survival of the soul after death and its ability to communicate with the living, swept the United States. Physicians quickly dismissed such notions, usually as simple fraud,[118] but occasionally as natural mental phenomena best explained by reference to such recognized biomedical concepts as Baron von Reichenbach's odylic force, phrenological neurophysiology, or W. B. Carpenter's doctrine of unconscious cerebration.[119] Popular enthusiasm for spiritualism seemed to decline in the late 1850s. Yet by raising questions as to the precise nature of an afterlife, a disquieting intellectual residue had been left behind, the investigation of which accelerated a revolution in psychiatric thought.[120] Bucke's fascination with a previously unknown form of consciousness was clearly a part of that process.

That spiritualism demanded serious scrutiny by certain middle-class intellectuals was suggested by several developments in the late 1860s and early 1870s. Though some prominent men of science such as John Tyndale, Thomas Huxley, and Michael Faraday scoffed at spiritualism, an impressive number of reputable scientists openly declared their belief. In the United States, as early as 1855, the highly respected chemist, Robert Hare, confounded his colleagues by affirming the validity of spiritualistic phenomenon, and he was joined the following year by John B. Fairbanks, the editor of the *Scientific American*. In the mid-1860s Alfred Russel Wallace, who, with Darwin, was the cofounder of modern evolutionary biology, publically affirmed that spiritualism explained far more of the esential human condition than did the concept of natural selection. In 1870 William Crookes, one of Britain's leading physical chemists, produced the first in his series of publications claiming a belief based on the empirical study of such phenomena as seances and thought transfer. And Oliver Lodge, perhaps preeminent by 1900 among English physicists, turned to spiritualism in the early 1880s.[121] The apostasy of such noteworthy scientists had not been convincingly and publicly refuted; indeed it seemed quite the reverse had taken place. In the United States, it is true, a committee of Harvard faculty had briefly investigated and then dismissed spiritualist claims in 1857. But far more disquieting was the report released in 1871 by the London Dialectical Society. A committee composed of some thirty professional men maintained a moderate but generally favorable disposition toward paranormal phenomenon.[122] By the early 1870s then, spiritualism appeared to be gaining a significant measure of scientific credence. It was within this context that prominent members of the Anglo-American psychiatric and neurological community launched a vociferous counterattack.

Prominent among those neuroscientists who derided spiritualism in the 1870s were the physiologist, W.B. Carpenter, neurologists W.A. Hammond and George M. Beard, and the alienist, Henry Maudsley. In contrast to spiritualists, who claimed to have identified a new power of the human mind, these individuals were wedded to a conception of mind that allowed little speculation as to the role of a dynamic unconscious.[123] Theirs was a far more static perspective which sought to explain the etiology of insanity largely by reference to the anatomical localization of discrete cerebral lesions. In milder mental disturbances the lesions were construed as functional rather than structural, but still centered at a specific anatomical site. Behavioral symptoms, the sole basis for commonly used classifications of insanity, were expressed in terms of disordered emotions, reason, or willpower, all static and mechanical notions of cerebral faculties. That a particular patient fell victim to a specific form of insanity was ascribed, in rigidly deterministic terms, to a malignant hereditary diathesis. Certainly unconscious cerebration was acknowledged and popularized as a variety of mental activity by Thomas Laycock and W. B. Carpenter, and Continental authorities such as Carl Gustav Carus and Edward von Hartmann had published works that suggested that the unconscious played a major role in the functions of the human mind.[124] But in general the notion of a dynamic unconscious as a potent source of mental activity and pathology was foreign to the alienists of the 1870s. Instead, most would have accepted Carpenter's notion that the control of mind ultimately rests with the will. It is a faculty by which the individual, Carpenter wrote,

can to a great degree *direct* his thoughts and *control* his feelings . . . and keep his appetites and passions under subordination . . . And in proportion as he does this, will he so *shape* his Cerebral mechanism (which, like all other parts of the organism, *grows-to* the manner in which it is habitually exercised).[125]

The will, in effect, became the prime determinant of both immediate behavior and permanent character. This notion was clearly resonant with the values that permeated the economic and political rhetoric of liberal individualism. If a deficiency of will might express itself in a social sense as cowardice, pauperism, or immorality, in neurological terms it vividly revealed itself as insanity.[126] For Victorian neurology, as for social theory generally, the essential capstone was the concept of individual volitional control.

If the spiritualist doctrines of unconscious powers of mind challenged specific aspects of neuroscientific orthodoxy, it struck equally at the social and intellectual authority of spokesmen for medical knowledge. It would not have escaped the notice of men like Maudsley that many of the exponents and most of the adherents of spiritualism in England were from the lower working class. As such, the doctrine represented on one level a class-based challenge to the hegemony of middle-class professionals.[127] On quite a different level, the debate revealed an interclass epistemological conflict. Medical psychology, of all the Victorian biomedical sciences, was the most closely wedded to an older metaphysical and, in some instances, theological tradition. As historians have argued, the Victorian conflict between science and religion was, in an important sense, a dispute less concerned with specific scientific theories than with the identification of legitimate sources of authority in matters of science. By 1870 laymen had displaced the clergy and their doctrines of natural theology, and put in their stead a positivist and secular epistomology as the exclusive foundation for valid science.[128] Because of its residual metaphysical linkages, medical psychology appeared particularly vulnerable to an attack from a revitalized religious source. Spiritualism, an intuitive, individualistic doctrine dignified by the support of eminent scientists such as Wallace and Crookes, posed just such an epistemological threat to recently secularized natural science and, especially, neuroscience.

The representatives of medical psychology, as a result, based their critique of spiritualism less on clinical grounds than on an argument concerning the nature of valid knowledge. Spiritualism was accepted only by "credulous folk" who are "incapable . . . of observing correctly"[129] or by university metaphysicians habitually "on the side of delusions."[130] Their testimony as to paranormal phenomena was worthless, according to Hammond, for such believers "have no clear conception of what knowledge is, and of how things are to be proved."[131] Rather, Beard argued, "only the testimony of experts can be of value," to which Carpenter, in an effort to exclude scientists such as Crookes and Wallace, added the qualification that the term experts was meant to imply only those trained in mental science.[132] Ultimately, only by strict adherence to the cannons of empirical method – "habits of accurate observation, and of correct reasoning upon the facts so learned" – rather than by faith based largely on intuitive perceptions would the fraudulent nature of spiritualism be clearly exposed.[133] Empiricism, these men hoped, would once and for all vanquish the pseudoscience of spiritualism as a challenge to the legitimacy of neuropsychiatric authority.[134]

It was precisely this empiricist challenge that ironically for these representatives of orthodox neuroscience, stripped spiritualism of its supernatural connotations and ensured its incorporation into the range of research interests encompassed by a new medical psychology. The major Anglo-American catalyst of this transformation was the Society for Psychical Research (SPR). Founded in London, England, in 1882 it included at times among its members such distinguished laymen as Tennyson, Ruskin, Gladstone, John Addington Symons, and Lewis Carroll. William James, Freud, Jung, Pierre Janet, and Cesare Lombroso all became corresponding members.[135] But two groups appear to have been particularly significant in its gestation and activities. The first were scientists such as Wallace, Crookes, and especially the physicists, Oliver Lodge, William Barret, and their less committed colleagues, J.J. Thomson and Lord Rayleigh. To Victorian physicists the spiritualist notions of survival after death or spirit communication must have seemed no less fantastic than the many newly discovered forms of energy such as cathode rays, and certainly highly compatible with their more traditional belief in amorphous ether, an all-encompassing universal substance which united both force and matter.[136] This mixture of apparently empirical yet antireductionist thought appealed equally to a second important group within the SPR. It had coalesced around the Cambridge moral philosopher, Henry Sidgwick, and included Arthur Balfour, Edmund Gurney, and Frederick Myers. Together these men, no longer able to accept Christianity, sought solid secular proof of a morally coherent and benevolent universe. They were affronted by the arrogance of traditional empiricists, to whom mind was an epiphenomenon of matter and questions of an after life legitimate only in a metaphysical context. As a consequence, they resolved to use the materialists' own weapon, to prove through empirical research the validity of the spirit world.[137]

The new organization must have struck a responsive cord, for by 1900 membership had grown to almost 1,000 while a decade earlier the American branch claimed nearly half that number including the Harvard physiologist, Henry Bowditch, and the psychologists, William James and George Stanley Hall.[138] That critical empirical evaluation had become the hallmark of the society's investigations was clear from its dismissal of most forms of physical mediumship – table rappings, levitations, spirit materialization – as shoddy pretense, in preference to the study of the far more sophisticated phenomena of telepathy and clairvoyance. This emphasis had two consequences. First, the professional mediums and the uncritical believers in supernatural events left the society by the end of 1886.[139] Secondly, the work of the society drew frequent favorable comment and serious attention from academic physicans and psychologists. At the International Congress of Experimental Psychology in 1889, for example, members of the SPR joined Charles Richet, the French physiologist, and a majority of the other delegates in arguing against a purely material basis for psychology. At such conferences, in the pages of the *Proceedings of the Society for Psychical Research,* and in other publications, the Society seemed to contemporaries to occupy the cutting edge of the new psychology. Pierre Janet joined the group because he discerned a kinship with his own studies on hysteria. Myers introduced the work of Freud and Janet to England and, in turn, particularly through his *Human Personality and Its Survival after Death* (1903), influenced Carl Gustav Jung, Alfred Binet, and Boris Sidis. Edmund Gurney's work on dissociated personality was, according to the American neurologist, Morton Prince, equal in stature to that of Pierre Janet.[140] In the late 1880s, then, the society, by deleting both trickery and the supernatural from spiritualism, had fashioned the intellectually respectable discipline of psychical research.

Many physicians and psychologists whose professional stature and doctrines were not inextricably linked to the older somatic paradigm were receptive to new perspectives on psychopathology. The work of the SPR on the dynamic unconscious was viewed by these disgruntled professionals with cautious but optimistic interest. Yet for orthodox medical psychology to accept openly notions of the unconscious required sanction from within medicine, an event which occurred, in a symbolic sense, in 1882. It was then that J.M. Charcot, Europe's premier neurologist, presented a paper on hypnotism to the Académie des Sciences in Paris. Though in academic circles hypnotic phenomena were generally regarded as no more legitimate than mesmerism, Charcot's interest in the topic had been stimulated by the French physiologist and psychical researcher, Charles Richet. Almost immediately his theories were revised by Hippolyte Bernheim and the Nancy School of hypnotism. But, significantly, hypnotism and the unconscious had gained virtually instantaneous medical respectability.[141] In France there were powerful political motives for this metamorphosis, but that the enthusiasm for the new field was similar elsewhere is clearly indicated by the rapid increase in the volume of medical publications devoted to hypnotism.[142] The new approach to psychotherapy claimed to tap the unconscious mind through the induction of a trance. It was a tactic that allowed physicians to deal with the mildly disturbed rather than, as the somaticists had done, concentrating attention on the floridly insane. This prospect attracted to Charcot's clinics a number of brilliant students – James, Freud, Janet, Binet[143] – many of whom also maintained ties with the English psychical researchers. Through their subsequent widely reviewed work, such as Janet's *Psychological Automatism* (1889), the notion of the unconscious became an essential dimension of a medical psychology in which the will played a vastly diminished role.[144]

If the neuroscientists of the 1870s rejected spiritualism and apparently allied notions such as hypnotism for reasons largely related to the issue of professional doctrine and authority, their colleagues a decade later, Bucke among them, were presented with no such difficulties. Spiritualism, stripped of its supernatural connotation by the empiricism of the SPR, had become psychical research at precisely the moment that Charcot and his followers legitimated the notion of a subconscious mental world. Acceptance of the new line of thought was not, of course, universal. In the United States, for example, George Stanley Hall withdrew from the SPR, accusing its members of an unscientific approach to psychology, and by 1898 only two American universities specifically engaged in psychical research apart from work in abnormal psychology.[145] Among American neurologists, interest in psychotherapeutics and the unconscious confronted what Nathan Hale has characterized as "belligerent somaticism" and few physicians beyond the urban Eastern seaboard regularly practiced hypnotism.[146] Yet during the 1890s even the traditional *American Journal of Insanity* devoted space to papers on hypnotherapy and subconscious ideation.[147] In part the receptivity to the new European doctrines may have derived from the work of what has been called the Boston School, an informal cluster of psychologists and physicians all of whom in their publications dealt with aspects of the unconscious. Among its members were neurologists Morton Prince and James Jackson Putnam, psychologists William James, Boris Sidis, and Hugo Munsterberg, and alienists Edward Cowles and Adolf Meyer. At least four of these men were members of the SPR and made little marked distinction between medical research on dreams or hypnosis and psychical investigations of telepathy and the survival of the soul. Indeed, James, who introduced Freud's work to America and stood preeminent among the first generation of American psychologists, when discussing "The Hidden Self" in *Scribner's Magazine,* appeared to group under the same heading phenomena ranging from faith healing to dissociated personality states.[148] Yet a professional medical audience could not have ignored the opinions of Putnam, first professor of the diseases of the nervous system at Harvard, whose work on posttraumatic neurosis led him, initially, to recognize the legitimacy of psychological causation and later, to actively engage in psychotherapeutic practices.[149] His friend, Morton Prince, professor of neurology at Tufts University, was a keen student of Charcot and Janet, whose work he followed in his popular *The Dissociation of a Personality* (1906). He was the founding editor, in 1906, of the *Journal of Abnormal Psychology,* while five years later Putnam became the first president of the American Psychoanalytic Association.[150] As Nathan Hale concludes, partly "through the work of Prince and Putnam the major foundations of a new psychotherapy were laid between 1885 and 1900."[151] Significantly, the premise upon which the new orthodoxy stood was the legitimacy of the newly discovered powers of the unconscious.

It is only by viewing Bucke's work within the context of late nineteenth-century psychiatry's debate over unqualified somaticism that the genesis of his *Cosmic Consciousness* becomes fully apparent.[152] The London Asylum library subscribed to the SPR's annual proceedings, beginning with the first volume in 1882, and Bucke's book, in turn, was found in the society's library.[153] In the work of an individual such as Frederick Myers, Bucke would have found psychological theories of the "subliminal self" in a congenial blend with metetherial notions of a world soul and optimistic declarations of faith in humanity's spiritual evolution.[154] Indeed, the cosmic sense was in many respects similar to the hypnotism, spiritualism, or telepathy that had occupied the attention of Myers and his English colleagues.[155] Of such allied phenomena, Bucke told the British Medical Association, the "labours of the Society for Psychical Research have made it to me plain these . . . really exist."[156] It was clear to him, he continued, that:

these are not cases in which outside agents are acting on or through a human being, but are cases in which a given human being has faculties which are not commonly possessed. Whether any given faculty, such as one of those now alluded to, shall grow, become common, and finally universal in the race, or wither and disappear, will depend upon the general laws of natural selection, and upon whether the possession of the nascent faculty is advantageous or not to the individual and to the race.[157]

In precisely the same manner, his analysis of cosmic consciousness was, he believed, "physiological as well as psychological" and the subject itself could "be studied with no more difficulty than any other natural phenomenon." There was nothing about the appearance of this new power of mind that was either "supernatural or supranormal – or . . . anything more or less than a natural growth."[158] Cosmic consciousness, in short, was precisely similar to the discovery of those other unconscious mental phenomena responsible for launching the revolution in late nineteenth-century medical psychology.

In the formulation of his ideas on mental pathology and the functions of the mind, Richard Maurice Bucke revealed, albeit in idiosyncratic form, his congruence with a major shift in psychiatric thought. At the same time as late-Victorian alienists endorsed a deterministic hereditarian view of insanity, a sizeable minority among them began an exploration of what would prove a far more malleable etiological notion, the dynamic unconscious. Degeneracy theory had been born of a heightened awareness of nineteenth-century class divisions, and the social authority accorded to psychiatry was a recognition of the profession's role in naturalizing in objective scientific terminology what was essentially a statement about class relationships. If the concept of degeneracy served an important function in exculpating alienists from blame for both low cure rates and the austere custodial character of asylums, it narrowed the focus of their attention to social deviants among the poor. They were rescued from this confinement by what was in essence a popular lay attempt to elaborate a new view of the mind – spiritualism – a doctrine that overtly challenged the fragile hegemony of neuroscientific orthodoxy. In quelling this attempt to democratize neurological theory with the weighty vocabulary of empirical science, psychiatry was forced to incorporate a new view of a dynamic unconscious, potentially at odds with traditional notions of the primacy of will. Almost unwittingly alienists gave birth to a concept that eventually would allow them, albeit in various theoretical guises, to transcend the confines of the asylum and to extend the authority of their medical gaze[159] to a middle class presumably free from hereditary taint.

5

Treatment tactics and professional aspirations

Implicit in the etiological notion of degeneracy was a profound therapeutic skepticism, for those unfortunates doomed to madness by hereditary taint appeared beyond the pale of efficacious medical intervention. In most Anglo-American asylums incarceration became an exercise in environmental management rather than active treatment. Yet by the end of the nineteenth century, attacked by their medical colleagues and themselves frustrated and discontent, alienists began a search for more aggressive therapeutic tactics. General medicine had rationalized its pharmacopoeia and introduced promising new treatments such as thyroid extract, while surgery, in the wake of antiseptic method, had catapulted to the forefront of medicine. Surely, alienists hoped, a comparable advance might be found for the keepers of the mad. Some, following Freud, sought such innovation in communication with the pathogenic unconscious. Others, more traditional, demanded psychopathic hospitals devoted solely to the aggressive care of acute, potentially curable cases, while the chronic insane would be relegated to custodial institutions. For still others, following the model of contemporaneous public health, prevention became the essential focus of psychiatry and was given practical expression in the mental hygiene movement.[1] Bucke's psychiatric career reflected exactly these therapeutic concerns. After a brief flirtation with aggressive treatment following his asylum appointment, he lapsed into therapeutic conservatism. Only in the final half-dozen years of his superintendency, inspired by both the criticisms and the example of general medicine and surgery, did he follow many of his alienist colleagues in a search for new and aggressive therapeutic strategies.

Bucke once conceded that as a novice superintendent his views on therapy bore an inverse relationship to his practical experience. By way of example, he may have had in mind his 1877 attack on masturbatory insanity. Described in medical literature since the mid-eighteenth century as the cause of a variety of somatic diseases, in the late-Victorian period leading alienists such as Henry Maudsley, Daniel H. Tuke, J. C. Bucknill, and Thomas Clouston assured their readers of the prevalence and validity of masturbatory insanity as a clinical entity, a view shared by many other physicians including the prominent American neurologist, Edward Spitzka.[2] With this authoritative testimony for support alienists and general practitioners experimented with therapies that ranged from benign dietary manipulation to radical surgical procedures.[3] Not until the close of the century was the causal nexus between masturbation and insanity disputed. Though many older alienists continued to endorse the legitimacy of the diagnosis, others, like Maudsley, accepted the opinions of a younger generation (among them Havelock Ellis), who saw masturbation as no more than a possible cause of neurotic disorders.[4] Yet, in its heyday, the masturbatory hypothesis had given physicians and patients a reassuring explanatory schema for poorly understood diseases,[5] and provided a vehicle for the expression of deeply rooted social anxieties. Autoeroticism was perceived, first, as the ultimately antisocial act, a denial of membership in an organic community aptly captured in the designation "the solitary vice." Secondly, masturbation represented a reckless squandering of precious resources, a wanton disregard for the concept of individual thrift and accumulation upon which the stability of nineteenth-century society depended. And, finally, "self-abuse" was an abnegation of will, a loss of the responsibility and self-control which, in the aggregate, had the potential to disrupt the social cohesion of modern civilization.[6] Antisocial, profligate, and disorderly, masturbation was the bodily analog of behavior abhorred by nineteenth-century middle-class society. It was within this context that physicians, Bucke among them, approached the insane masturbator with a sense of cleansing vengeance. Eliminating these moral degenerates, in effect, represented a symbolic sacrifice to the fragile goals of social cohesion, economy, and order.

Bucke began his attack on self-abuse in March of 1877 by adopting a surgical procedure devised by Dr. David Yellowlees of Glasgow for the insertion of a silver wire through the foreskin of the penis.[7] "I . . . intend to give this operation . . . a fair trial in the course of the next six months," he optimistically confided to his journal, "there is no doubt that if a plan could be hit upon of stopping this vice 'mt' a great many cases could be relieved or cured which are now hopeless."[8] Initially he "carefully selected cases as belonging to a class in which the habit seemed to some extent a cause of the insanity." A twenty-five-year-old clerk, for example, was operated upon after it was recorded that he seemed "very dull and stupid when admitted, whole appearance indicated a masturbator." This enigmatic selection criteria becomes more intelligible from an examination of the case records for the nineteen patients upon whom the "wiring" procedure was performed, and the two additional patients who were simply circumcised. The majority were in their early twenties and all but one were single, both characteristics that distinguished them from a random sample of all male inhabitants of the asylum. Most were laborers or farm employees, few were known to have had a family history of mental illness, and four had previously experienced psychiatric problems. A dozen patients were said to suffer from mania, four from melancholia, three were imbeciles, one was demented, and one had no diagnosis.[9] In only one instance, a case of sodomy, was a punitive connotation openly attached to the procedure.[10] It would seem, then, that the ideal case was a young, single, working-class male who suffered from mania. It was no coincidence that to precisely this type of individual bourgeois society had come to attribute the potential for dissolute and disorderly behavior.

The surgical treatment was evaluated by Bucke in his annual report for 1877. As a result of extensive technical difficulties, including patient opposition and postoperative infection, eight patients were wired twice and three underwent three procedures.[11] Unfortunately, the outcome did not appear to justify the effort and Bucke reported complete failure in almost half his cases. In fact, the casebooks reveal an even more depressing record. Of the twenty-one patients upon whom procedures were done, two showed "marked" improvement, three were said to demonstrate "slight" improvement, and the rest remained unchanged.[12] Bucke now qualified his earlier view of the solitary vice. "Whether it is ever the sole cause of insanity I very much doubt," he conceded, though he continued to believe that in some patients the practice might "assist in bringing on the attack," while other cases were "aggravated by this habit." In terms of treatment however, he was forced to admit "that in only a small proportion of all those cases in which masturbation exists could removal of the habit, even were this possible, be expected to be of any benefit to the patient."[13] Not even the surgeon's knife, it seemed, could eliminate the masturbatory social evil. In the end, only revoking the disease status of masturbation provided a permanent end to what had once been construed as a virtual epidemic.

Faced with the failure of his aggressive approach to masturbatory insanity, Bucke lapsed quickly into therapeutic conservatism. The psychiatric journals and textbooks that he and his assistants consulted provided little to inspire revision in this approach to treatment. In addition to the *American Journal of Insanity* and the *Journal of Mental and Nervous Diseases,* the small asylum library contained works by Krafft-Ebing, Bucknill and Tuke, Lombroso, and Ferri, in all of which the dominant theme was therapeutic pessimism.[14] The accuracy of such views was confirmed by statistics. In Britain, for example, a scant 7.7% of patients in county and borough asylums in 1870 were assumed to be curable, an estimate that was barely exceeded by actual discharge figures.[15] For acute cases there was, both Bucke and the Inspector of Asylums concluded, some hope of recovery.[16] But in such cases, cautioned Bucke, " 'cure' means spontaneous recovery, more or less aided by management, but seldom, if ever, actually brought about by medical interference." Those cases that did not rapidly remit were rooted in a hereditary taint, for which the prognosis was hopeless. Indeed, Bucke conceded, "Insanity is essentially an incurable disease." The only chance of "decreasing the aggregate amount of lunacy" lay in the vague hope of prevention.[17]

The treatment programs of the London Asylum that resulted from this pessimistic view of lunacy were succinctly summarized by an appreciative patient in a letter to a local newspaper:

Very little medicine is given or required. They depend on regular hours, avoidance of excitment, good diet, in many cases complete rest, in others regular exercise in the open air, and for those who are strong enough, regular employment, a moderate amount of amusement, combined with firmness and kindness in their management, for all cures.[18]

It was a description of therapy that tallied closely with several published by Bucke.[19] Like the British authorities, Bucknill and Tuke, he was convinced "that the treatment of disease of the mind resolves itself into an endeavor to place the whole physical system on the best possible basis of health and efficiency." With this objective accomplished, nature healed the curable while the residual cases, the majority, in fact, joined the "ranks of 'Chronic Insanity'."[20] This philosophy of passive therapeutics was congruent with both the prevailing government parsimony which proscribed expensive alternatives, and with a lengthy tradition in Anglo-American psychological medicine.

Bucke's approach to mental therapeutics had distant roots in the *traitement moral* described in English translation by Philippe Pinel in 1806 and applied independently, with seeming success, by Samuel Tuke, a Quaker layman, at the York Retreat.[21] It represented a disavowal of physical therapies, including bleeding and the administration of drugs, in favor of a psychological approach. Ideally, the stricken patient was quickly removed from his or her home to the calm of a small, isolated institution staffed by numerous empathetic but firm attendants. Under their watchful and reasoned guidance, the lunatic was given distracting work, a sound diet, gentle amusements, and religious instruction. The exciting cause removed, the physical lesion in the brain slowly healed.[22] Aspects of the method were slowly adopted in some English asylums in the wake of the revelations by the Select Committee on Madhouses in 1815, though some, such as Dr. William Lawrence of Bethlem Asylum, dismissed the "moral pharmacopoeia" as worthless.[23] Such reluctance may have reflected an implicit awareness on the part of physicians that laymen were equally qualified to direct the application of moral therapy. As well, the method was modeled on circumstances that were considered unobtainable at the large, understaffed pauper asylums. As a result, by the mid-1840s only five county asylums in England had abandoned mechanical restraint. In the following decade, perhaps more confident after reading of the successful experiences of Robert Gardiner Hall and John Conolly, an increasing number of Anglo-American superintendents did away with the more obvious restraining appliances and adopted the philosophy of work, amusements, and religion.[24] It was in some respects a short-lived triumph, for restraint reappeared in the 1860s but the gospel of work and religion lived on.[25] Indeed, the survival of the latter two management tactics as a pale shadow of moral treatment points to what lay at the philosophical core of the system. It was "no kindness for kindness's sake" but, rather, "was designed to encourage the individual's own efforts to reassert his powers of self-control."[26] To be sure, moral therapy was more humane than earlier techniques, but beneath its rhetoric it sought to replace external restraint with the force of internalized values derived from work, prayer, and appropriate recreation. Patients controlled in this manner were ultimately less difficult to manage then those requiring constant coercion, and were certainly more compatible with the sensibilities and social expectations of their keepers. It was, as Bucke so correctly realized, simply a matter of gaining "moral ascendency" over his charges.[27]

At the London Asylum, few drugs were given for psychiatric indications. Magnesium sulphate was used to treat seizures, while opium, potassium bromide, and chloral hydrate served as sedatives.[28] But as far as promoting a cure for the mental disease of his patients, Bucke wrote, "I do not believe that drugs are capable of taking any part in the attainment of that end."[29] His expenditures on pharmaceuticals reflected this belief, comprising in 1887 0.6% of the annual cost of individual patient maintenance. This figure was comparable to that of other asylums in Ontario, suggesting that his therapeutic practices were similar to those of his Canadian colleagues.[30] Indeed, in only one area was the use of drugs at the London Asylum controversial. In contrast to Bucke, for example, the Superintendent of the Toronto Asylum, Daniel Clark, was convinced of the therapeutic efficacy of alcohol.[31] The disagreement between Clark and Bucke mirrored a wider debate that had raged in England during the 1860s over the physiological actions and the nutritional value of alcohol. It was a debate that initially concerned the nature of physiological evidence and later found itself swept into the issues raised by the evangelical temperance movement.[32] A number of prominent neuroscientists such as W.B. Carpenter or Bucknill and Tuke drew analogies between the effects of intoxicants and states of cerebral pathology. Undoubtedly the most ardent British advocate of medical temperance in the late 1870s was Bucke's friend,

Benjamin Ward Richardson.[33] It was at his suggestion, Bucke acknowledged, that he began his campaign to remove alcohol from the London Asylum.[34]

His first expression of doubt as to the value of alcohol appeared in print in 1879, and by 1882, after initially discontinuing the use of beverages in favor of pure spirits, he terminated all prescriptions for alcohol.[35] After five years of this policy Bucke felt he could document not only a large financial saving, but also a decline in deaths and an increase in the cure rate. He attempted to explain, in neurochemical terms, the rationale behind his findings. The nerve molecule, he argued, is composed of atoms which collapse during activity to liberate energy and which are rebuilt at rest. Because in "size the alcohol molecule is to the nerve molecule about as 1 to 100" and "probably, a thousand times as hard," when the two collide the latter is "crushed, bruised and broken." The liberated nerve force is first evident in an imbiber as exhilarated behavior, but when all energy has been dissipated, a state of insensible intoxication is reached. Precisely the same mechanism accounts for the effects of chloral hydrate or morphine which, like alcohol, can penetrate the brain tissue. In fact, the degree of intoxication from these various compounds, Bucke argued, correlated directly with the molecular size of the substance, thereby confirming his theory of colliding molecules.[36] It was a style of argument, blending organic chemistry in a mechanical framework with neurohistology, that revealed the influence of Benjamin Ward Richardson's earlier research on anesthetic agents.[37] The vocabulary of cerebral chemistry in which it was expressed gave the argument a tone of objective authority unavailable to the moral advocates of abstinence. As the Inspector realized, "Dr. Bucke's testimony . . . is particularly valuable . . . as he is not generally known as a 'temperance man' . . . nor indentified [sic] with the so-called temperance movement." His views, "arrived at upon entirely professional grounds without references to the moral or economic aspects of the question" were, therefore, particularly compelling.[38]

Less controversial than Bucke's disavowal of alcohol was his endorsement of the nonrestraint approach to asylum management. Despite the rhetoric of moral treatment, few public asylums managed to do away with restraint, and it was not-infrequently viewed as a positive therapeutic tool.[39] Bucke himself wrote in 1877 of nonrestraint that "I do not believe it can be or ever was practised" and endorsed the judicious use of mechanical appliances, especially crib beds, as effective and inexpensive.[40] Though Inspector Langmuir concurred, his successor, Dr. W.T. O'Reilly, was an ardent champion of nonrestraint and to him Bucke politely gave credit for its adoption at the London Asylum.[41] In fact, however, the disenchantment with the use of restraint appears to have antedated O'Reilly's appointment in 1881. In his 1879 report, Bucke argued that, although some patients always required physical control, in general "the use of restraint makes restraint necessary." This insight he attributed to his assistant, Dr. Beemer, who, though working in the refractory ward, found many patients when released from restraint to be cooperative and harmless.[42] Previously, Bucke wrote, "it used to be thought the correct thing to do to strap the violent patients in restraint chairs, lock them in rooms, secure their hands in muffs, or confine them in a crib." In 1880, the number of patients subjected to restraint was ninety-three, a figure that was almost halved two years later. As well, an *open-door system* was adopted in 1883, despite the earlier reservations of Inspector Langmuir, so as to give the majority of patients free access to the asylum grounds.[43] A year later, Bucke reported, "during the last fifteen months, we have not used at this Asylum any mechanical restraint or seclusion." Professing himself surprised at the success of the approach, he denied that there had been an accompanying increase in the use of chemical sedation. The efficacy of the nonrestraint he attributed to two factors. First, the ability of an attendant "to gain moral ascendency over the patient" replaced mechanical appliances with the constraints of personal authority and social conventions. Secondly, and of greater importance, was "the employment of the patients."[44] In the asylum, more than elsewhere, it seemed that idle hands were truly the devil's playground.

In his first annual report, Bucke, claiming that "suitable employment is found for every patient fit to work," suggested that such activity was among the most efficacious "remedial agents" available to the alienist. A decade later it had become for him, as for many contemporary asylum superintendents, "the best of all therapeutic agents at our command."[45] In 1884, for example, over 84% of patients were employed on an average day, an increase of 27% over the preceeding year, which Bucke attributed in part to

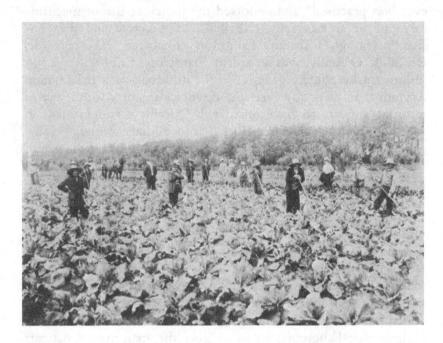

Figure 13. Patients working on the London Asylum farm, n.d.
Source: London Psychiatric Hospital.

discontinuing the use of restraint. Of almost 900 patients, no more than 70 did not work and, of these, 50 were physically incapable. Males assisted the institution's maintenance men, tended the farm and garden (Figure 13), and worked in the laundry or kitchen. Female patients engaged in sewing or knitting, cleaned the wards, or helped in the laundry and dining rooms.[46] To induce patients to work, Bucke wrote, "all means short of compulsion . . . are used; privileges are given to patients who work, and withheld from those who do not." The recalcitrant were sent with working parties and eventually, despite their initial reluctance, joined in the task assigned. By preoccupying the patient with employment, Bucke believed, the need for mechanical restraint or constant supervision was removed, the patient's mind focused "on realities" rather than "morbid thoughts," and the tedium of asylum life was ameliorated. No doubt for some patients escape from the confined wards did exert a positive therapeutic effect. Concurrently, working patients diminished certain institutional expenditures, a fact appreciated by the Inspector, who urged maximum productivity from the asylum's inhabitants.⁴⁷ Cast in the guise of treatment, patient employment was calculated both to obscure the therapeutic impotence of the physicians and to alleviate the escalating cost of the asylum. It was assumed by the system's proponents that the will, under the discipline of work, would regain control of the disordered mind. In this process, reality, expressed in terms of regularity, obedience, self-control, and productivity, was the active therapeutic ingredient. It was a notion that would surely have had a familiar ring to those many Victorians familiar with the oft-quoted gospel of work.⁴⁸ Indeed, in many respects the London Asylum had come to resemble a very large workhouse.

All work and no play, however, made patients less amenable to treatment. Without relief from wards and work they became, Bucke wrote, victims of "the horrible torpor and langor that unless prevented, inevitably tend to settle on asylum life, and develop [sic] it in darkness second only in intensity to the grave itself." For that reason, he believed amusement ranked next to work "as a curative agent."⁴⁹ It was a term that comprised a number of activities, many of which must have come as welcome diversions to the patients. They were entertained at weekly concerts at which local groups such as the Seventh Fusilier Band or the Pall Mall Street Church choir supplemented the music provided by the asylum orchestra under the direction of the bursar, Dr. Sippi. Alternatively, appropriately light selections were provided by the Asylum Dramatic Club (Figure 14), events in which the families of the medical officers usually participated, and Bucke himself recited poetry during variety evenings. These occasions, together with weekly dances and occasional illustrated lectures, must have been welcomed by the resident medical staff as much or more so than by the patients. But attendants needed constant encouragement to participate and a system of fines was imposed for those who failed to appear at concerts or dances.⁵⁰ These events provided not only a forum for charitable acts by local organizations, but also permitted such groups a quick glimpse at the strange world of the asylum. Some activities, in fact, took the lunatics out among the sane populace, a presence which local newspapers did not fail to notice. Trips to a visiting circus or the London fall fair were common, and the "Asylum Eleven" (Figure 15) traveled to nearby cities to compete in

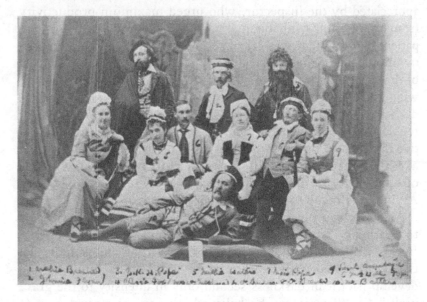

Figure 14. London Asylum Drama Group, c. 1885. Source: R. M.
Bucke Collection, University of Western Ontario.

cricket matches.[51] Asylum entertainments, then, ostensibly designed as therapy, also broke the institutional tedium for the
medical staff and their families and gratified both philanthropic
urges and the curiosity of local citizens.

Employment and amusements were joined in Bucke's approach to therapy, as in many late nineteenth-century asylums,[52]
by religion. Of ministers he wrote, "My own opinion is that
their services are as important to the welfare of the patients as are
those of the attendants or the doctors."[53] Though Bucke's own
theological views never returned to the orthodox Christianity of
his early childhood, he eventually accepted the existence of both
a Divinity and an afterlife.[54] His hostility to organized religion
had clearly dissipated by the late 1870s and in his 1880 report he
pleaded that the absence of an adequate chapel led the list of
"most pressing wants" at the asylum. On one occasion, in fact,
he himself was forced, since no minister was available, to read
the sermon.[55] An appropriate hall was eventually built and Protestant clergy of various denominations held Sunday-morning
services in rotation, while Roman Catholic services were con-

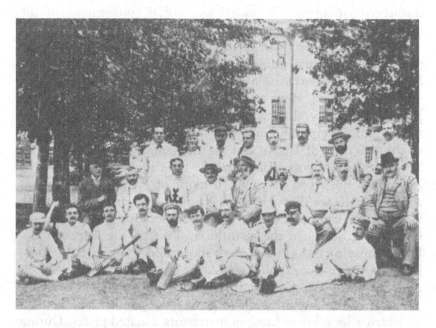

Figure 15. London Asylum cricket team, 1895. Source: London Psychiatric Hospital.

ducted every second Sunday afternoon. Attendants were urged to participate and were restricted in their activities until services were concluded. Initially, Bucke's policy regarding patients was equally coercive. "Sunday morning service is attended by all the patients who are well enough to go," he wrote, "No one is allowed to remain absent from service because he or she does not want to attend." A decade later, for reasons never made explicit, the compulsory approach had been discontinued and less than half the patients chose to attend.[56] Though Bucke was silent on the benefits he anticipated from religious services, given his own agnosticism, it seems safe to conclude that they were less theological than behavioral. Regular chapel attendance was both a form of routine, in itself considered beneficial to the mad, and a social activity calculated to distract the patient from introverted preoccupations. The morbid thoughts that characterize lunacy would be, if not displaced, at least challenged by the uplifting spiritual messages preached by the visiting clerics. Religion, then, was perceived as a means of reorienting the disturbed patient to the moral and social conventions of the external world.

The treatment protocol of the London Asylum, based on the triumvirate of work, religion, and constructive amusement, was both typical of most Anglo-American institutions and consistent with a pessimistic view of etiology and prognosis. But this approach to therapy also had a subtle role beyond the confines of the asylum. The public, indeed, had many opportunities to learn of the practices of Bucke and his assistants. "Our Western Fair has begun in London," Bucke wrote to Walt Whitman, "and the Asylum is full from morning to night of people to see friends and people to see through the institution." During the fair week in 1877, for example, as many as 600 spectators daily filled the halls and grounds of the institution. Though the Inspector believed most of the visitors were motivated by "morbid curiosity," the open-door policy was continued until after Bucke's death in 1902.[57] Other members of the public encountered the practices of the asylum while attending the popular athletic days to which a long list of London merchants donated prizes. During the winter entertainment season, a constant flow of small groups such as orchestras, church choirs, or amateur theatrical companies spent evenings in the asylum. To such visits were added tours by the grand jury, local politicians, and visiting medical gatherings.[58] By word of mouth and in print, some of these groups conveyed their impressions to the literate and interested middle class.[59] More accessible to the general public were the frequent laudatory newspaper accounts describing asylum entertainments, athletic events, additions to the physical plant, or the productivity of the farm. Not all newspaper portrayals, of course, were favorable to the asylum. Bucke was disturbed by what he viewed as the sensationalism favored by one of the local papers. For example, a not-untypical headline proclaimed: "Death in Bath Tub, Horrid Fate of a Lunatic at the Asylum, Fatally Scalded While Taking a Bath."[60] Such stories, when balanced against the more frequent favorable accounts of the asylum's progressive treatment program, betrayed the ambivalence of public attitudes toward insanity. The insane were portrayed as potentially violent and unpredictable, whereas, under appropriate care, they became tractable proof of the efficacy of society's humane ministrations. Indeed, the treatment given at the asylum raised no significant public debate, for it was, in an important sense, a display case in which Victorian society saw itself.

That the Victorian public would have found the principles of lunacy therapy not only acceptable, but also familiar is hardly surprising. The goal of treatment, Bucke observed, was "not so much the cure of disease as . . . the re-humanization of the patient." In the process drugs played no part; rather, it was a routine of "regular work, amusements, [and] properly ordered mental exercise" which defined the return to human status.[61] In effect, the products of successful treatment embodied the Victorian ideal of good citizenship while at the same time reinforcing that model as behavior best calculated to reverse the ravages of madness. Abstinence was a virtue, whereas its alternative was, quite literally, the first step to insanity. Religion, even when the worshipper attended as a result of compulsion, was less a means of imparting theological doctrines than a mode of conveying standards of socially acceptable behavior. Above all other values stood work. Bucke considered it "about the best thing in the world for either the sane or the insane man."[62] Under its constraints, as in society itself, physical force was rendered unnecessary, and all were compelled, by group pressure or material rewards, to participate. In fact, cure was defined in general as the integration into the social practices of the asylum, whether religious services or entertainments, and in particular, by the patient's productivity.

Reason, in short, was social conformity and productive behavior; its converse, madness. The equation was derived from the ethos that underlay Victorian society and, in turn, it served to reinforce that paradigm. Industrial capitalism had little time for eccentricity, preferring instead citizens both conventional and diligent. That such behavior represented reason, and lunacy its abandonment, was as much the covert message of the alienists as it was the overt philosophy of Samuel Smiles. If degeneration theory had served to justify existing class relationships by equating poverty and madness, asylum treatment advertised the rules of correct conduct by which the fate of both the lunatic and the pauper could be avoided. Together psychiatric theory and practice made starkly explicit the values of Victorian society, deriving authority from the pervasive nature of that social paradigm and, in turn, conferring authority through the imprimatur of objective science.

The treatment practices of Anglo-American alienists of the 1870s were not only congruent with prevailing social theory, but in their therapeutic pessimism they shared, as well, an important affinity with general medicine. Many physicians of this period subscribed to a profound skepticism about the utility of medicines when compared to the inherent healing power of nature. This ancient belief was reformulated in modern guise by the clinicians of the Paris School during the early nineteenth century and perpetuated by their descendants to whom Bucke was exposed as a postgraduate student. It was a message that was introduced to America in the 1830s in such works as Jacob Bigelow's *Discourse on Self-Limited Diseases* (1835) and Elisha Bartlett's later study, *An Essay on the Philosophy of Medical Science* (1844). The movement gained momentum during the 1860s and reached a symbolic climax in 1863 with Oliver Wendell Holmes's hotly debated address to the Massachusetts Medical Society, "Currents and Counter-Currents in Medical Science," in which he urged pharmacological caution upon his colleagues.[63] To an extent he was preaching to the converted, for by the 1860s among orthodox practitioners the worst excesses of heroic therapy, especially copious bleeding and large doses of calomel, had already been substantially modified. In fact, a not-insignificant number of physicians were sympathetic to homeopathic practice, with its infinitesimal dosages. Drugs were certainly not abandoned, but they were now intended largely as symptomatic adjuncts to nature's dominant role.[64] Yet if pharmaceutical skepticism, as the example of Sir William Osler suggests, continued into the twentieth century, the shrill tones of the debate over what Holmes referred to as "the nature-trusting heresey" faded rapidly in the 1880s.[65] Medicine had begun to purge itself of traditional pharmacological follies and now groped toward what were perceived as more rational and efficacious therapies.

Unfortunately for psychological medicine, the discipline could marshal no etiological or therapeutic innovations comparable to those in other specialties. The 1880s brought general medicine a new understanding of bacterial diseases and an introduction to endocrine therapy, while surgery reaped the benefits of the new antiseptic orthodoxy. But alienists remained burdened with the impotence of the increasingly dated therapeutic conservatism that they had so recently shared with most other physicians. In North

America the increasing obsolescence of asylum medicine was dramatically underscored by the turbulent relationship between alienists and a new group of practitioners who, with experience gained with nerve injuries during the Civil War, claimed specialized knowledge of neurological disorders. They constituted themselves the American Neurological Association in 1875 and founded the *Journal of Nervous and Mental Disease* in which to publish their work. Though the majority of papers appearing there dealt with organic neurology, a few prominent neurologists such as William A. Hammond and Edward Spitzka wrote monographs on insanity.[66] In part this reflected the neurologists' varied clientele. Many emotionally disturbed patients fell short of the criteria necessary for the only other form of psychiatric care – asylum admission – and, instead, were treated as private outpatients for *neurasthenia* by physicians such as George M. Beard or subjected to the *rest cure* by Weir Mitchell and his followers. More significant, however, was the impact of the German approach to nervous diseases. There, as the careers of Wilhelm Griesinger or Theodore Meynert suggested, no sharp distinction was drawn between psychiatric and neurological practice. And above all, the German model stood for a rigorous scientific method.[67]

It was, in fact, on the issue of science that in 1877 American neurologists launched a spirited attack on the alienists. Instead of keeping abreast of and contributing to medical science, charged Edward Spitzka, asylum superintendents could be relied upon to publish little more than "crude pathology and administrative generalities."[68] The virulence of the neurologists' assault diminished after 1882, but their point had been made and it reinforced an impulse toward reform already evident among the alienists themselves. At the 1881 annual meeting of asylum superintendents a call was heard for a more vigorous and scientific approach to institutional treatment. Over the ensuing decade the older alienists who had devoted their academic papers to administrative issues were displaced by younger men, especially the assistant physicians recently admitted to the organization, who directed discussion toward current therapeutic topics. By 1890 this trend was sufficiently advanced for the president of the superintendents' association to feel secure in calling for a reorganization of the group so as to incorporate both the lessons of modern neurology and the career interests of younger alienists.[69]

It was against this background of changing conviction that the senior American neurologist of the period, Weir Mitchell, was persuaded to address the superintendents' meeting in 1894. He initially refused, making clear his critical stance, but eventually agreed to undertake what he later described as the "most distasteful task of a varied life." His sweeping critique made two basic points. First, the "cloistral lives" of the asylum physicians not only encouraged "certain mental peculiarities," but also ensured their "isolation from the mass of the active profession." Often political placemen, these physicians assumed the "absurd label of 'medical superintendents' " and slipped into chronic medical lethargy.[70] Secondly, as neurologists had long argued, alienists were foolish to assume that they could be at once "farmers, stewards, caterers, treasurers, business managers and physicians." The worst consequence of such "stupid folly" was a lack "of competent original work," despite an immense reservoir of pathological material.[71] "We commonly get as your contributions to science," Mitchell continued, "odd little statements, reports of a case or two, a few useless pages of isolated post-mortem records, and these sandwiched among incomprehensible statistics and farm balance sheets."[72] In effect, Mitchell condemned his audience as isolated administrators devoid of any scientific or medical acumen. Yet far from taking offense at his charges, the alienists greeted his onslaught with a standing ovation. The only critical responses at the meeting suggested that Mitchell's comments were already so widely accepted as to be redundant, while the *American Journal of Insanity* later offered nothing but favorable editorial comment. Indeed, the very decision to invite Mitchell, having been forewarned of his views, suggests that he was preaching to the converted.[73] Asylum superintendents were engaged in a desperate search for scientific legitimacy; only by modernizing their doctrines and treatments could their specialty be rescued from chronic professional obscurity.

Bucke was clearly sensitive to the precarious status of alienists in the eyes of both fellow physicians and, increasingly, the general public. There was, he felt, a popular stigma attached to individuals confined to asylums. He joined with his fellow superintendents in Ontario in petitioning the Inspector to change the designation of their institutions from asylums to hospitals. The former, the alienists argued, was popularly associated with "barbarous treatment" by which "few recoveries were affected," while the latter implied rapid cure through "all advanced scientific appliances and methods."[74] But Bucke himself went well beyond these semantic debates in an idiosyncratic attempt to prove both the efficacy and the modernity of asylum practice. The etiological concepts he deployed and the status problems they were expected to redress were common to all alienists; it was the manner in which Bucke acted upon his theory that set him apart from his colleagues. Where the quest for professional stature was soon to lead other alienists to champion the creation of psychopathic hospitals, to support the mental hygiene movement, or to endorse psychoanalysis, for Bucke it led in quite another direction. In February of 1895 he launched his second program of aggressive therapeutics: the use of gynecological surgery to cure mental disease.

The physiological theory upon which Bucke based his surgical enthusiasm was rooted in views widely held by nineteenth-century physicians. Years earlier Bucke had explained the special status of the genitalia in terms of the sympathetic innervation that connected them to the brain. It was a theme to which his co-worker, Dr. A.T. Hobbs, returned, asserting, "the brain is intimately connected with the uterus and its appendages through the great sympathetic system and . . . disturbances of the latter are reflected upon the former." This phenomenon, he later elaborated, occurred "reflexly or sympathetically." The belief that pathology in a specific organ might manifest itself in the abnormal function of a distant area of the body, a process termed *sympathy*, dated from classical medicine. But it was the description of the reflex arc in the 1830s by Marshall Hall and Johannes Müller that at last appeared to provide experimental evidence of the neurophysiological mechanism by which reflex sympathy likely occurred. The concept of reflex, though in Hall's work restricted to unconscious actions integrated in the spinal cord, was extended by Thomas Laycock to the complex activities of the cerebral hemispheres.[76] The doctrine of reflex action rapidly became an accepted mode of explanation in the standard textbooks of physiology by W. B. Carpenter or R. B. Todd and William Bowman.[77] It was now possible for those concerned with mental pathology to attribute a variety of disorders to disturbances elsewhere in the body in a manner schematically indistinguishable from the ancient doctrine of sympathy, yet couched in the sophisticated vocabulary of reflex physiology.[78] In fact, though convinced of the etiological validity of what J. C. Bucknill and Daniel H. Tuke referred to as "Insanity by Sympathy,"[79] Henry Maudsley conceded the hybrid nature of the concept in his authoritative work on mental pathology. Of the notion that "the mind might be deranged by disease in other parts of the body" he wrote,

perhaps *sympathy* was as good as seeming explanation of these effects as the modern doctrine of *reflex action* . . . So many and various are these pathological and physiological reflex actions that we shall perhaps for the present do best to embrace them under the wide term – sympathy.[80]

Until the final years of the nineteenth century most physicians were willing to accept Maudsley's advice.[81]

In the late nineteenth century the concept of reflex action found frequent application as an explanation for the alleged connection between the brain and pelvic disease in women. Medical students learned from W. B. Carpenter's discussion of mental physiology that "a functional disturbance of the cerebrum is often induced by the irregular action of other parts of the nervous system, especially those connected with the reproductive apparatus."[82] This view was given particular clinical expression in the textbooks of two specialties. Both English and American gynecological authorities argued that irritations in the pelvis were transmitted, via the sympathetic nervous system, to the brain and were manifested as syndromes which ranged from mild neuroses to florid insanity. For the interested practitioner a number of monographs were available devoted to specific aspects of psychogynecology, notorious among them, Isaac Baker-Brown's defense of his widely condemned clitoridectomies.[83] Similarly, clinical applications of reflex action were common in the work of prominent psychiatrists. Bucknill and Tuke, for example, argued that second only to intemperance among physical causes of insanity were "epilepsy, and disorders more or less connected with the uterus." Henry Maudsley expanded on this notion that "the uterus and its appendages . . . not infrequently play an important part in the production of insanity." Pelvic disorders, he explained, caused a general diminution of nerve "tone" in the predisposed woman which resulted in "disordered emotion." This functional disturbance, if prolonged, produced "actual nutritive change" in the brain and eventually the "structural disease" associated with chronic insanity.[84] American alienists such as Edward Jarvis and Isaac Ray found little to dispute in the gynecological opinions of their British psychiatric colleagues. As well, the neurologist Weir Mitchell conceded the importance of pelvic disease in case of hysteria and his colleague, Edward Spitzka, asserted in 1889 that menstrual irregularities were a proven cause of severe mental disorder.[85] No informed practitioner of the late nineteenth century could help but conclude that pathology in the female generative organs was intimately linked to aberrations in the function of the central nervous system.

Despite this extensive body of medical theory upon which to base gynecological treatment, the surgical program at the London Asylum had a largely fortuitous origin in the arrival in 1895 of A. T. Hobbs, a newly appointed assistant physician with an interest in pelvic surgery.[86] Previously Bucke had expressed skepticism that gynecological surgery might cure epileptic insanity and the treatments used at the Asylum for such incidental gynecological problems as came to the attention of physicians were largely conservative local measures such as pessaries or carbolic acid dressings.[87] The results of the first months of surgical intervention, however, changed doubt to cautious optimism. Though 2 of the initial 19 patients died, all those remaining recovered physical health and twelve allegedly showed recovery or improvement in their mental symptoms. Another 15 cases with similar results quickly followed, but Bucke, in discussing his work at the 1896 gathering of asylum superintendents, remained circumspect. He admitted that the mental cures, with time, might prove "evanescent" and that any surgical procedure, not solely gynecological operations, might have a positive influence on the mental condition of the insane.[88] But despite these reservations, the volume of surgical cases continued to grow, with an average of 42 operations in each of the ensuing five years. While there were five deaths among these 209 patients, the vast majority recovered from their physical disease and an average of 64% annually were said to show mental recovery or improvement[89] (Table 5.1). These consistently positive results swept away the reservations Bucke had initially expressed. By

Table 5.1 *Yearly reported results of gynecological surgery at the London Asylum, 1895–1900.*

Year	Physical outcome				Mental outcome			Dead
	Number of cases	Recovered	Improved	Unchanged	Recovered	Improved	Unchanged	
1895	19	11	6	0	3	8	6	2
1896	27	14	7	2	2	13	8	4
1897	46	46	0	0	14	21	11	0
1898	41	41	0	0	12	12	17	0
1899	40	39	0	0	14	14	11	1
1900	55	55	0	0	17	16	22	0

Sources: O.S.P., 1896, 44–5; 1897, 82–5; 1898, 44–51; 1899, 76–81; 1900, 73–5; 1901, 36–40.

1899, the surgical work, begun "in quite a tentative manner" with "considerable doubt," had become simply "a matter of course" at the London Asylum.[90]

Though the London physicians claimed throughout their surgical program that the operations, in Hobbs's phrase, "were not performed with a view to curing the insanity of these patients,"[91] it is clear that the objective of simple gynecological rehabilitation was rapidly replaced by that of psychiatric recovery. The results from the first nineteen cases convinced both physicians that mental improvement had occurred in 63%. Such an unusual therapeutic response must have been irresistible to alienists frustrated by the norm of chronicity. It had always been an axiom of asylum practice that, in Bucke's words, "the treatment of diseases of the mind resolves itself into an endeavour to place the whole physical system on the best possible basis of health."[92] But the success of the pelvic surgery reinforced the more specific belief that "in some cases, at least, the insanity rests upon the utero-ovarian disease and may be cured by the removal of this." It was no accident, Bucke argued, that among all the procedures, those designed to remove diseased ovaries, to cure disorders of the cervix, or to restore a healthy endometrium revealed the greatest efficacy. These three anatomical areas were "the most vital . . . organs of the female sexual system" in which, "in fact, centres the life of the woman as such."[93] Almost from the beginning of their work, then, the London alienists entertained the suspicion, as Hobbs wrote to Bucke, that the operations would likely "aid in the mental recovery" of insane women.[94]

Armed with promising initial results and an apparently valid theoretical basis for their work, Bucke and Hobbs plunged into gynecological surgery with enthusiasm. According to Hobbs, 93 of the first 100 women patients examined were found to have pelvic disease, while by 1900, 85% of patients examined had a positive diagnosis. He implied that as a result of his initial findings a larger number of female patients were examined, usually under anesthesia, but gave no indication as to how the women were selected. Indeed, he explicitly noted that the insane neither experienced nor reported symptoms as did normal women, nor were they easily examined. Bucke simply commented that, "We have naturally examined those cases in which there seemed the greatest likelihood of finding disease."[95] At least three factors may explain why Bucke and Hobbs appear to have had difficulty finding gynecological disorders among their patients. First, in a period in which obstetrics remained a relatively crude and often expensive discipline, many of the working-class women in the asylum may have borne the scars of a traumatic delivery.[96] Secondly, in the early twentieth century venereal disease was widespread and led to significant pelvic pathology. At particular risk for contracting infections were sexually active women, that is, married women in the twenty to sixty age category, the group from which most of the London Asylum's surgical patients were drawn.[97] Finally, many conditions such as retroversion and retroflexion of the uterus, later recognized as normal variations, were considered pathological states by Victorian gynecologists.[98] It seems likely, as Bucke claimed, that 10% of the London Asylum's female patients may have suffered from either real or perceived pelvic disease.

Since a review of published work by Bucke and Hobbs fails to make readily apparent their specific selection criteria, data was gathered on 228 surgical patients and compared to 173 age-matched patients who did not undergo surgery.[99] The mean ages of the groups were 36.4 ± 9.9 (SD) and 37.2 ± 11.4 (SD) years, respectively. It might have been assumed that those only recently afflicted with psychiatric illness and without personal or family history of such disorders would appear attractive surgical candidates. However, the duration of attack prior to institutionalization was almost identical in the two groups, nor was there, in those patients for whom data was recorded, a difference in the number of previous admissions or the frequency of a family history of psychiatric disease. Those patients who were foreign-born or from minority religious faiths might have been expected to have had their social marginality reflected in increased vulnerability to surgical treatment. However, both groups of patients were divided in similar fashion between Roman Catholics and Protestants and a comparable proportion – 72% for the surgical patients and 69% for the control group – had been born in Canada. To explore the possibility that surgery carried a punitive connotation, the mode of admission was compared. Warrant patients were those deemed a clear threat to society, yet both surgical and control groups revealed similar proportions of patients admitted by this method. Nor could the two groups be differentiated on the basis of recorded misbehavior while in the asylum. Suicide attempts, escapes, and the use of restraint occurred with equal frequency in both groups.

A more revealing line of inquiry concerns mental and physical symptomatology. The patients undergoing surgery were most likely to demonstrate agitated behavior and less likely to be delusional ($P < .005$) than were control patients. This suggests that the nonoperative patients experienced a more severe form of psychiatric disturbance and were recognized to have a less favorable prognosis. While symptoms of gynecological disorders, such as pain, discharge, or abnormal bleeding, were recorded relatively infrequently, surgical patients were significantly ($P < .005$) more likely to have such problems mentioned in their case notes (16%) than were control patients. At the time of admission, a significantly greater ($P < .01$) number of the surgical patients had their mental symptoms assigned to puerperal circumstances or sexual activities such as masturbation or nymphomania, though the number of such diagnoses represented a small portion (12%) of the total admissions. At the time of admission, then, a rough triage must have occurred principally on the basis of behavioral characteristics but taking into account gynecological symptoms and presumptive etiology. That a rapid initial screening process likely occurred is borne out by the haste with which surgical patients underwent their operations: 50% had been treated within two months and 70% within six months of admission.

The sorting process was further expedited by taking into account parity and marital status. Despite the similarities of age, religion, and place of birth, a significantly ($P < .005$) greater number of surgical patients were married than was the case with control patients, and surgical patients were more likely ($P < .005$) to have had children. That many surgical procedures were related to injuries most likely sustained during childbirth is given added credence by a review of the diagnoses. Laceration of the perineum and of the cervix constituted the primary diagnosis in 14% and 13% of cases, respectively, while 30% of the diagnoses were for a subinvoluted or prolapsed uterus. A certain portion of the remaining 43% of diagnoses, which included hypertrophied cervix and endometritis, may have had a similar obstetrical ori-

Table 5.2. *Gynecological disorders diagnosed*

Primary diagnosis			Secondary diagnosis	
N	Percentage	Condition	N	Percentage
0	0	None	80	35
29	13	Endometritis	16	7
68	30	Subinvolution/prolapsed uterus	32	14
33	14	Lacerated Perineum	10	4
29	13	Lacerated cervix	13	6
6	3	Hypertrophied cervix	12	5
15	7	Retroverted or retroflexed terus	20	9
31	14	Tumor	1	0
17	7	Other/unknown	44	19
228	101		228	99

gin (Table 5.2). The case selection process at the London Asylum, then, favored married women in their midthirties who had borne children and who did not reveal delusional symptoms known to be associated with a poor psychiatric prognosis (Table 5.3). In short, Bucke and Hobbs chose as their patients individuals who likely combined presumptive pelvic pathology with a reasonable hope of mental recovery.

The surgical results reported on an annual basis suggested a very positive therapeutic response. These statistics from 226 cases Bucke summarized in his final report: four patients had "died as a result of the operation"; "nearly all the rest" recovered physically; and 149, or 66% of patients recovered or improved mentally. That these patients would not have shown mental recovery without surgical intervention was suggested by contrasting the female recovery rate for 1890–5 of 37.9% of admissions to the 52.7% during the next half-decade of gynecological work. During this ten-year period the male recovery rate did not change.[100] That at least some of Bucke's cases may, indeed, have owed their psychiatric recovery to their surgical experience seems possible. As many as the one-third of patients, predicted by current literature, may have simply responded to the placebo effect associated

Table 5.3. *Characteristics of gynecological and age-matched control patients, London Asylum, 1895–1900*

	Surgical group (N= 228)	Control group (N= 173)
Mean age on admission (years)	36.4 ± 9.9	37.4 ± 11.4
Duration of attack before admission (months)	22.4 ± 41.3	22.6 ± 44.8
Known previous admissions	35 (15%)	17 (10%)
Known family history	49 (21%)	40 (23%)
Canadian birthplace	165 (72%)	120 (69%)
British Isles birthplace	40 (18%)	29 (17%)
Protestant	193 (85%)	134 (77%)
Roman Catholic	30 (13%)	36 (21%)
Admitted by warrant	37 (16%)	34 (19%)
Delusional behavior on admission	134 (59%)	136 (79%)[a]
Married or widowed	165 (72%)	74 (43%)[a]
Known children	70 (31%)	31 (18%)[a]

[a] $P < .001$

with any surgical procedure. Secondly, individualized care, such as was given only to surgical patients in the asylum, is acknowledged by contemporary psychiatric literature to exert a significant positive influence on the prognosis of institutionalized patients.[101] There are, then, plausible reasons for assuming that Bucke's favorable figures may have had some validity.

A comparison of the case notes for operative patients and age-matched controls fails to substantiate Bucke's therapeutic claims. Though the records at the asylum were frequently incomplete or uninformative, an attempt was first made to describe the postoperative course of the surgical patients. Of the 228 patients identified, 18 months postoperatively 46% were improved or recovered physically, 6% had died, and no physical data was recorded for the remaining 47%. When the mental condition of the patients was assessed from the case notes after the same time lapse, only 48, or 21%, were improved or recovered (Table 5.4). Secondly, when the discharge figures of the surgical and control patients were compared, no significant

Table 5.4. *Postsurgical course of gynecological patients*

	Physical				Mental			
	At 6 mos.		At 18 mos.		At 6 mos.		At 18 mos.	
	N	%	N	%	N	%	N	%
Improved or cured	69	30	105	46	75	33	48	31
Unchanged or worse	3	1	2	1	28	12	69	30
Dead	8	4	14	6	8	4	15	7
Unrecorded; lost to follow-up by discharge	148	65	107	47	117	51	96	42

Table 5.5 *Discharge status of gynecological and control patients*

	Recovered/ improved		Unchanged/ worse		Unknown		Died	
	N	%	N	%	N	%	N	%
Control patients	78	46	13	7	1	0	80	46
Surgical group	118	53	14	6	4	2	87	39

difference between groups was found in terms of the number of patients sent home as recovered or improved or the number who died at the institution. Among the surgical group 39% died and 53% were discharged as recovered or improved, while for the control group 46% represented the proportion in both categories (Table 5.5). Thirdly, five years after discharge, 5% of discharged control patients and 7% of surgical patients had been readmitted to the London Asylum. Finally, and perhaps most revealing, is a comparison of the duration of hospitalization for the two groups. The mean duration of stay for the control group was 83.8 months ± 134.6 (SD) from the date of admission. Surgical patients, in contrast, remained in hospital 117.0 months ± 164.5 (SD) from admission and 94.5 months ± 142.7 (SD) from the date of their surgical procedures (Table 5.6). These figures, then fail to document a positive psychiatric response to gynecological intervention. Indeed, based on duration of stay, it would appear that surgical patients had a worse prognosis than did age-matched controls.

Table 5.6. Duration of stay for gynecological and control patients

	0–12 mos.		13–24 mos.		25–120 mos.		121 + mos.		Mean ± SD (months)
	N	%	N	%	N	%	N	%	
Control patients	77	46	16	10	37	22	37	22	83.8 ± 134.6
Surgical group	86	40	22	10	44	20	64	30	117.0 ± 164.5

With the benefit of hindsight it is possible to demonstrate statistically the failure of Bucke's surgical program. But his alienist contemporaries had no such advantage; moreover, they accepted his views on the reflex action of genital pathology, as well as his desire to enhance the status of asylum medicine, two shared convictions that might have predisposed them to acknowledge the validity of his argument. But it is clear that this was not the case. Methodological weakness was one objection marshaled by those among Bucke's alienist colleagues who opposed his surgical program. Dr. James Russell of Hamilton argued that "all such statistics which are published prior to a two years' test of their efficacy are comparatively worthless," while Dr. Daniel Clark of Toronto demanded a trial of regular and surgical treatments for comparable groups of patients. If some patients recovered, Russell argued, it was due entirely to the increased care associated with any type of surgical procedure. Bucke, in reply, denied that (after four years of surgery) his follow-up period was too brief. As well, in none of the fifty-one patients upon whom nongynecological operations had been performed had significant mental improvement been noted, thereby negating the notion that better nursing care alone explained his results. Russell complained, too, of the lack of objective proof of pelvic disease in many patients and attributed the alleged findings to a "relentless surgical fury" on the part of gynecological enthusiasts. Bucke and Hobbs countered that their diagnoses were always independently confirmed by a physician unconnected with the asylum. Buttressing all these methodological criticisms was a smoldering sense of moral outrage. To Russell the gynecology represented "the wholesale surgical mutilation of helpless lunatics," while to Clark the work "of these raiders of feminine reserve" was an affront to woman's innate sense of modesty. Confronting these charges, Bucke replied that "we never operate without the consent of the patient's friends, and . . . the patient's physician is always consulted and . . . he is always asked to be present." The real moral censure, Bucke and Hobbs concluded, should be reserved for those who attempted to deny to insane women the benefits of essential gynecological surgery that were made readily available to the sane.[102]

In 1897 Hobbs complained of the "bitter opposition" aroused by the London surgical work and Bucke, in his penultimate annual report, vastly understated the case when he lamented that the gynecology proceeded "without much encouragement from our fellow alienists."[103] The Ontario government, on the advice of "certain doctors," likely Russell and Clark, refused financial support for the project. The Inspector of Asylums fought openly with Bucke, asserting, "The general and unlimited examination of females . . . would . . . destroy all their finer sensibilities, and prostitute, even among the insane, all the elevating moral fibre of their being."[104] Nor was opposition confined to Bucke's Ontario colleagues. Certainly some other Anglo-American alienists had also acted upon the compelling logic of reflex action to launch gynecological programs. George H. Rohe of Maryland was the leading North American exponent during the 1880s, and others echoed his views.[105] Still other physicians, such as Ernest Hall of Vancouver, long after the last procedure in London, continued to attack reflex insanity through operative treatment.[106] But the vast majority of alienists remained unmoved by the obvious therapeutic implications of an etiological concept that most of them in general endorsed. In 1891 Dr. I. S. Stone of Washington, himself an exponent of psychogynecology, sent an inquiry to twenty "representative asylums" in the Eastern and Midwestern states. Of eighteen respondents, only three believed that many cases of female insanity were due to pelvic pathology. Six years later Dr. Russell of Hamilton surveyed "120 of the principal alienists in Great Britain and America," discovering that all but three superintendents believed less than 5% of their female cases were due to pelvic disease, and very few endorsed gynecological intervention.[107] That operative gynecology had a place in psychiatric therapeutics was a notion viewed with skepticism by the 1896 gathering of American asylum superintendents, and openly denied at the 1897 meeting of the British Medical Association. Few physicians, it appears, were willing to risk the earlier and celebrated fate of Isaac Baker-Brown, the British exponent of clitoridectomy for relief of insanity, by pursuing reflex physiology to its logical therapeutic conclusion.[108]

Far from retreating in the face of this barrage of criticism, Bucke proposed in 1897 that all asylum gynecological work in Ontario be centered in London where appropriate instruments and trained nurses were already available. In support of his position he enlisted several outside forces. On the day following his centralization proposal the London *News* carried a very favorable account of surgery at the asylum, while several days earlier the London Medical Association passed a resolution endorsing his gynecological program and urging increased government support.[109] In November of that year Bucke sent a circular to 350 doctors in Western Ontario, describing ninety-two surgical cases, of which 65% allegedly recovered mentally, and inquiring if the physicians felt the work should continue. Not surprisingly, given the phrasing of the letter, only 2 of the 255 respondents opposed the gynecological surgery.[110] Bucke made these results public in 1898 and shortly afterwards solicited support from an important and vocal group, the National Council of Women. Apparently at the instigation of the London chapter, the Council circulated a resolution to local chapters which urged greater government support for Bucke's surgical activities. Commented the acerbic Dr. C. K. Clarke of the Kingston Asylum, "The wonder is that these dames, being decidedly 'non compos' at the time they drew up their remarkable petition, did not call in the enthusiastic young surgeon to attend to their cases."[111] Despite these vigorous attempts to defend and extend the surgical program, with the retirement of Hobbs in December of 1900 and Bucke's accidental death shortly after, the gynecological era at the London Asylum met an abrupt demise.

There is no evidence to suggest that Bucke's gynecological program was founded on a gender-based hostility toward female patients. Though he was an intimate friend of two literary figures, Walt Whitman and Edward Carpenter later widely known as homosexuals, Bucke himself was heterosexual and there is no evidence that this surgery was a manifestation of deeply rooted anxiety about personal sexual indentity.[112] Nor was the surgery simply a professional cloak by which a Victorian physician expressed a general cultural antagonism toward women.[113] Certainly, Bucke shared the common sexual stereotypes of his generation. But he applied the physiological theory underlying these views with the same rigor to his male masturbators as to his gynecological patients. Moreover, as the violent opposition to his surgery on the part of alienist colleagues suggests, there was no necessary link between Victorian views of female psychosexuality and support for gynecological intervention. A more plausible explanation for his work lies in the threatened status of asylum medicine. For Bucke and Hobbs the attraction of gynecology lay primarily in its potential to provide a means by which alienists might modernize and legitimate the authority of psychological medicine.

This rationale for his gynecological tactics was clearly expressed in Bucke's 1898 presidential address to the American Medico–Psychological Association. He warned his audience that only with the adoption of modern therapies would alienists be seen as credible consultants, specialists in their own field of psychiatric disorders. A year later his younger colleague bluntly aserted;

Let not some alienists forget that they are living in modern times, and that every branch of scientific art is advancing. It will not suffice to hold up their hands and deplore the increase of insanity and the overcrowding of our asylums. The world will demand of them an account of what they are doing to increase efficiency in their methods and increase their ratio of recoveries.[114]

Fortunately, according to Bucke, "the immense strides recently made towards perfection in surgical procedure" offered hope to the alienists. Indeed, continued Hobbs, "No section of surgery had made more rapid strides towards perfection than that pertaining to the amelioration of the condition of women suffering from pelvic diseases." Compared to the "nauseating extracts, attenuated toxines and doubtful serums" of "non-progressionists," the gynecological treatment of insanity was an obvious "scientific advance." It was the "Rip-van-Winkle ideas" of conservative alienists that allowed "misery, discomfort, and disease to hold sway." By rejecting "medieval methods" in favor of modern surgical techniques, alienists would gain a respected place in the medical mainstream.[115]

The London physicians were correct that their gynecological techniques were among the most recent innovations in surgery. Until the antiseptic revolution in the early 1870s, operative gynecology remained a minor addendum to the larger field of obstetrics. The change that accompanied Listerism was captured by a gynecologist who observed at a meeting of the American Medical Association in 1882, "The peritoneal cavity is no longer the *terra incognito* of the surgeon, nor its invasion attended with the fears or dangers of even a very recent period."[116] With antisepsis, the practice of gynecology had reached, in effect, its take-off point. The American Gynecology Society was founded in 1876, the first textbook of gynecological pathology appeared in 1868, and an increasing number of general hospitals made provision for gynecological services. In London, England, only four hospitals had gynecological wards before 1862, while in the period from 1876 to 1888 another six opened such facilities. Similarily, the general hospitals in Montreal, Kingston, and Toronto all appointed attending gynecologists between 1883 and 1895.[117] Gynecology as an organized specialty was a very recent creation when Bucke and Hobbs launched their surgical therapeutics in 1895.

If the institutional superstructure of gynecology was of recent origin, so too were the procedures upon which this autonomous identity was based. In 1856 George Lyman reported finding only 300 cases of ovariotomy, the procedure done in 8% of the London cases, in the world literature, while 117 English hospitals performed only 22 such operations in 1863. Yet Spencer Wells alone, between 1864 and 1880, performed 800 ovariotomies, Lawson Tait reported 100 cases between 1880 and 1882, and, in the United States, Robert Battey became an evangelist for the many benefits of his "normal ovariotomy."[118] The diagnosis of cervical hypertrophy was introduced to gynecology in 1859 and two years later J. Marion Sims described a procedure for amputation of a lacerated or elongated cervix. His technique was modified over the next decade by a number of successors, including Dr. C. Schroeder, whose method Hobbs employed in 16% of his patients.[119] For uterine retrodisplacement and prolapse the pessary period came to an abrupt end with the introduction of Alexander's suspension operation, a procedure used at London in almost one-quarter of the cases, in 1881.[120] Finally, though the first successful abdominal hysterectomy was performed in 1853 and though numerous vaginal methods appeared subsequently, removal of the uterus, accounting for one-tenth of the London cases, remained rare until the late 1880s [121] (Table 5.7). As they argued, then, most of the operative techniques that Bucke and Hobbs adopted were products of the post-1870 antiseptic revolution. Through modern gynecology, in effect, alienists could leave behind the traditional stigma of therapeutic impotence to participate instead in the most spectacular innovations of Victorian medicine.

Table 5.7. *Principal gynecological procedures*

	N	%
Dilatation and curettage	48	21
Perineal repair	32	14
Cervical amputation	36	16
Uterine suspension	54	24
Hysterectomy	20	9
Ovariotomy	18	8
Other/unknown	20	9
	228	100

For those physicians among their audience who remained un-convinced that psychogynecology was validated by trends in modern surgery, Bucke and Hobbs offered a second, more ab-struse and rather more innovative line of reasoning. To account for the beneficial psychic effects of the operations, especially in cases of ovarian disease, Bucke wrote, "it seems to me that the recent physiological theory of so-called internal secretions will furnish the clue we want." Citing the example of "testicular juice," he argued that disease would result from either an absent secretion or a pathologically altered fluid which became "a toxic agent of unknown but probably great virulence."[122] Without abandoning reflex action as an equally likely explanation for the cerebropelvic nexus, Bucke and Hobbs associated their surgical work with what was clearly the most exciting development in late nineteenth-century physiology. Reflecting on this period Edward Schafer, perhaps the most prominent turn-of-the-century British physiologist, later observed, "The Old Physiology was based . . . on *nervous regulation;* The New Physiology is based on *chemical regulation.*"[123] The nerve impulses of reflex physiology, by analogy with the common electrical current, seemed familiar and readily comprehensible to even the most ill-informed practitioner. But to fully understand the concept of internal secretions demanded a grasp of such new and esoteric specialties as biochemistry.[124] By deploying endocrinology as a source of legitimation for his psychogynecology, Bucke at-tempted to place his work in a prestigious and specialized realm beyond the judgmental competence of the average practitioner.

This was an astute tactic, for it assumed that his professional contemporaries, though ignorant of the details of endocrinology, would be sufficiently familiar with the general concept to respect the scientific validity of his work. It was not an unreasonable assumption. The aging but eminent French neurologist, C. E. Brown-Séquard had focused international attention on internal secretions in 1889 with descriptions of the rejuvenation studies in which he had used injections of testicular extract. If his well-publicized announcement was enthusiastically greeted by quacks only too anxious to profit from dubious organotherapy, it also stimulated medical interest in glandular extracts. Perhaps most dramatic was G. R. Murray's successful treatment of thyroid deficiency in 1891 using an extract of sheep thyroid. Three years later Edward Shafer reported that dramatic cardiovascular effects of adrenaline and several investigators used extracts of the pancreas in a series of unsuccessful attempts to treat diabetes.[125] For clinical medicine such endocrinological developments seemed to hold immense therapeutic promise. Though no dramatic innovation had been made in pharmacology in the nineteenth century at all comparable to the achievements of surgery, tissue extracts might have been expected to help redress this deficiency. Even more important, however, was the role that internal secretions might play as an explanatory metaphor. The timeworn and vague concept of reflex action could soon be cast aside as an explanation for poorly understood disease in favor of the enigmatic but seemingly more scientific doctrine of internal secretions. By the end of the nineteenth century, then, the time seemed imminent when glandular secretions would yield important information on the cause and treatment of human disease. To frustrated alienists such as Bucke, this etiological and therapeutic progress must have appeared as a welcome means by which asylum practice could be integrated into the mainstream of nineteenth-century medicine.

Bucke had received his medical education during the heyday of therapeutic nihilism. Armed with these beliefs, and buttressed with the etiological dogma of degeneration, he revealed the therapeutic pessimism shared by most Anglo-American alienists. During the 1880s, however, this approach to treatment grew increasingly less congruent with the optimistic attitudes of general medicine and surgery. It now appeared that psychologi-

cal medicine was to become the backward specialty in an otherwise evolving profession. This fear sent alienists on a desperate
quest for progressive treatment techniques. If Bucke's own
search was idiosyncratic in content, it was also highly consistent
with the theories and professional ambitions of most other
alienists. Yet it was an approach doomed to failure. The development of the very gynecology he endorsed cast the notion of
pelvic insanity into disrepute, while the notion of reflex action
fell victim to increasingly sophisticated neurological knowledge
and new theories of endocrine regulation. The rejuvenation of
psychiatry, in fact, was not to occur at least until the First
World War, when shell shock cases and intelligence testing
created a pressing demand for expertise in psychological medicine.[126] Only then would Victorian doctrines of degeneracy and
somatic pathology finally fade as many psychiatrists, armed
with the notion of the dynamic unconscious, ventured beyond
asylums to seek both a new clientele and an expanded social
authority in the wider community.

Epilogue

Richard M. Bucke lived out his professional life in a time of turmoil for psychological medicine. Like his fellow students in North America and Europe during the 1860s, he was educated in a tradition of therapeutic conservatism. Aggressive surgery promised only a septic demise for the patient, while pharmaceutical intervention had at best the potential for fortuitous symptomatic relief. In clinical practice medicine's role was ordinarily confined to accurate diagnosis and prognostication. In a more general sense, medicine occupied itself in a search for etiological clues that would lead to a more efficacious therapeutics. Yet, paradoxically, this apparent medical humility coexisted with another and much more confident attitude, a conviction Bucke shared with many of his professional contemporaries. Scientism, often in the specific guise of positivism, provided an optimistic, secular epistemology by which representatives of Victorian science and medicine justified their claim to authority in fields encompassing both the natural and the social sciences. Empirical investigations, not metaphysical speculation or revealed religion, gave certitude to the knowledge necessary to guide science and society in a progressive fashion and, significantly, stature to those who provided that guidance.

Late nineteenth-century psychiatry, of all medical fields, best illustrated the ambiguity of therapeutic pessimism and positivist optimism. It was a discipline possessed of few cures but a great deal of weighty theory. A variety of British thinkers, especially Herbert Spencer, Alexander Bain, and John Stuart Mill, attempted to make of psychology a natural science, a notion entirely consistent with the neurophysiology elaborated by W. B. Carpenter. If the complex theorizing was done by a select few, Anglo-American alienists were only too willing to adopt this secular view of mind (expressed in the authoritative vocabulary of associationist psychology and cerebral localization) as the substratum for their own particular interest, mental pathology. Discussion of the mind to these physicians was a medical, rather than philosophical, topic and, so defined, assumed the same seemingly value-neutral quality that attached to other branches of science.

In particular, etiological notions of psychopathology were enunciated with a sense of dogmatic assurance. Borrowing from evolutionary biology, a number of psychotheorists, ranging from Cesare Lombroso to Hughlings Jackson, gave detailed form to the concept of mental degeneracy. Expressed with clinical detachment and based on accepted natural science, the theory appeared to provide an objective and accurate explanation for the discouraging prospects of asylum inmates. Yet the popularity of the theory cannot be accounted for simply on the basis of the authority of the science upon which it was apparently based. Rather, degeneration theory owed its appeal less to medical credibility than to its ability to explain and naturalize certain disconcerting realities of late nineteenth-century society. The inhabitants of public lunatic asylums were known to come from the working-poor and pauper class. Yet these patients were also defined by physicians as neurological degenerates. Poverty and degeneracy, in effect, were two sides of a very warped and inferior coin, a coin that was quite without value in the marketplace of industrial capitalism. In its congruence with – indeed, support for – Victorian class relationships, psychological medicine found the key to its social authority.

Judged as nature's misfits, most asylum patients were considered to have little hope of cure. After all, an inherited neuropsychiatric taint could not be expected to respond to even the most aggressive treatment. The resulting therapy was characterized by a custodial pessimism conducted in the most economical manner consistent with public sensibilities. Degeneration theory, in other words, justified the character of psychiatric care and treatment. It was only gradually that the alienists came to realize that custodialism carried with it unwelcome and unintended professional consequences. Not only were they and their assistants shut up in the same monotonous and oppressive institutions as their patients, but further, this very seclusion consigned them to an ignominious backwater of the medical profession. With the introduction of antisepsis, surgery marched ahead, and general medicine, by 1890, could point with anticipatory pride to the potential of the newly discovered internal secretions. But alienists remained confined and isolated in asylums, which, until the 1880s, had seemed imposing testimony to both public benevolence and the theoretical acuity of psychological medicine.

In an effort to transcend their narrow institutional confines, alienists adopted a variety of tactics. Some argued that prevention alone could deal adequately with inherited disease, a belief Bucke shared, and gave enthusiastic backing to the mental hygiene movement. Other alienists urged the creation of psychopathic hospitals dedicated to the aggressive medical treatment of potentially curable cases. It was in support of this concern for modernized, acute therapy that Bucke advocated gynecological surgery for certain of his female patients. Psychiatry, he felt, by adopting this approach would benefit and gain stature from the most recent developments in surgery and endocrinology. Finally, still other alienists followed European theorists such as Pierre Janet and Sigmund Freud in positing the existence of a covert but treatable unconscious as the source of most psychopathology. Bucke's speculations on cosmic consciousness, if idiosyncratic, were firmly anchored in the late-Victorian fascination with the dynamic unconscious.

Of all the professional options considered by alienists, the exploration of the subconscious mind was by far the most promising. If mental illness was the result of the unconscious gone astray in an otherwise normal person, the focus of psychiatry was suddenly expanded beyond a concern for the overtly mad and degenerate among the poor. And as the psychiatric gaze widened to encompass ostensibly sound and healthy middle-class citizens in the community, so too did the social authority of the profession escalate. Indeed, but for his accidental death in 1902, Bucke might well have lived to see psychiatry move beyond the asylum and become the professionl group exclusively charged, in the twentieth century, with the ultimately more intractable task of interpreting man to himself. In this new paradigm of mind, he would have been surprised to learn, the once-orthodox somatic idiom of Victorian psychiatry plays little significant role.

NOTES

Introduction

1. Thomas Hankin, "In Defense of Biography; the Use of Biography in the History of Science," *History of Science* 17, no. 3 (1979):3; Susan Reverby and David Rosner, "Beyond the 'Great Doctors' " in their edited *Health Care in America: Essays in Social History* (Philadelphia, Pa.: Temple University Press, 1979), pp. 3–16.
2. There are some exceptions to this statement. Gerald Grob's, *Edward Jarvis and the Medical World of Nineteenth-Century America* (Knoxville, Tenn.: University of Tennessee Press, 1978) views his subject's psychiatric career as secondary to his work with the federal census. Nancy Tomes's, *A Generous Confidence: Thomas Story Kirkbride and the Art of Asylum Keeping, 1840–1883* (New York: Cambridge University Press, 1985) is an excellent example of biographical social history.
3. Roy Porter, review of William Coleman, *Death is a Social Disease: Public Health and Political Economy in Early Industrial France* (Madison, Wis.: University of Wisconsin Press; 1982), *Times Higher Education Supplement* 11 March 1983, p. 22. A fine illustration of Porter's opinion is Michael MacDonald's perceptive study of Richard Napier, *Mystical Bedlam, Madness, Anxiety, and Healing in Seventeenth-Century England* (New York: Cambridge University Press, 1981).
4. The best general narratives of Bucke's life remain James H. Coyne, "Richard Maurice Bucke—A Sketch," *Proceedings and Transactions of the Royal Society of Canada* 2nd series, 12 (1906): 159–96; and Edwin Seaborn, "Richard Maurice Bucke, M.D., F.R.S.C., Professor of Nervous and Mental Diseases," in his *The March of Medicine in Western Ontario* (Toronto: Ryerson Press, 1944), pp. 290–307. Others of this genre include R. D. Walter, "From Comstock to Cosmic Consciousness," *JHMAS* 13, no. 2 (1958): 260–3; Cyril Greenland, "Richard Maurice Bucke, M.D., 1837–1902: A Pioneer of Scientific Psychiatry," *Canadian Medical Association Journal* 91, (22 Aug. 1964): 385–91; idem, "Richard M. Bucke, M.D., 1837–1902: Psychiatrist, Author, Mystic," R. M. Bucke Memorial Society for the Study of Religious Experience, *Proceedings of the First Annual Conference* (1965): 1–17; George Stevenson, "Bucke and Osler: A Personality Study," *Canadian Medical Association Journal* 44 (Feb. 1941): 183–8.
5. S. E. D. Shortt, "The Myth of a Canadian Boswell: Dr. R. M. Bucke and Walt Whitman," *Canadian Bulletin of Medical History* 1, no. 2 (1984): 55–70; Artem Lozynsky, *Richard Maurice Bucke, Medical Mystic: Letters of Dr. Bucke to Walt Whitman and His Friends* (Detroit, Mich.: Wayne State University Press, 1977). Other studies of Bucke and Whitman include Edmund G. Berry, "Dr. Bucke, Whitman's Canadian Friend," *Manitoba Arts Review* 4, no. 2 (1944): 5–13; Stanley E. McMullin, "Walt Whitman's Influence in Canada," *Dalhousie Review* 49, no. 3 (1969): 361–8; Harold Jaffee, "Richard Maurice Bucke and Walt Whitman," *Canadian Review of American Studies* 2, no. 1 (1971): 37–47; James Doyle, "R. M. Bucke," *Canadian Literature* no. 83 (Winter 1979): 201–6.

6. The major source on Bucke as a mystic is James R. Horne, "Cosmic Consciousness – Then and Now: The Evolutionary Mysticism of Richard Maurice Bucke" (Ph.D. dissertation, Columbia University, 1964). See also his "R. M. Bucke: Pioneer Psychiatrist, Practical Mystic," *Ontario History* 59, no. 3 (1967): 197–208; Brian Lauder, "The Two Radicals: Richard Maurice Bucke and Lawren Harris," *Dalhousie Review* 56, no. 2 (1976): 307–18; John Robert Colombo, "A Doctor of Mysticism: Richard Maurice Bucke," *Canadian Theosophist* 41, no. 6 (1961): 133–9; Cyril Greenland, "Richard Maurice Bucke, M.D., 1837–1902: The Evolution of a Mystic," *Canadian Psychiatric Association Journal* 11 (April 1966): 146–54; Leslie Armour and Elizabeth Trott, "The Self-Transcendence of Reason, and Evolutionary Mysticism," in their *The Faces of Reason, An Essay on Philosophy and Culture in English Canada, 1885–1950* (Waterloo, Ontario: Wilfrid Laurier Press, 1981), pp. 361–87.

7. The best accounts to date of Bucke's psychiatric career are Wendy Mitchinson's, "R. M. Bucke: A Victorian Asylum Superintendent," *Ontario History* 73, no. 4 (1981): 239–54; idem, "Gynecological Operations on Insane Women: London, Ontario, 1895–1901," *Journal of Social History* 15, no. 3 (1982): 467–84; idem, "Gynecological Operations on the Insane," *Archivaria*, No. 10 (Summer 1980): 125–44; Cheryl Krasnick, " 'In Charge of the Loons': A Portrait of the London, Ontario Asylum for the Insane in the Nineteenth Century," *Ontario History* 74, no. 3 (1982): 138–84; Rainer Baehre, "From Pauper Lunatics to Bucke: Studies in the Management of Lunacy in Nineteenth-Century Ontario" (M.Phil. thesis, University of Waterloo, 1976). Other sources include George H. Stevenson, "The Life and Work of Richard Maurice Bucke: An Appraisal," *American Journal of Psychiatry* 93 (March 1937): 1127–50; Cyril Greenland, "The Compleat Psychiatrist, Dr. R. M. Bucke's Twenty-five Years as Medical Superintendent, Asylum for the Insane, London, Ontario, 1877–1902," *Canadian Psychiatric Association* Journal 17 (Feb. 1972): 71–7; idem, "Three Pioneers of Canadian Psychiatry," *Journal of the American Medical Association* 200 (5 June 1967): 833–42.

8. The making of nineteenth-century psychiatrists has received little scholarly attention. See, however, Constance McGovern, " 'Mad Doctors': American Psychiatrists, 1800–1860," (Ph.D. dissertation, University of Massachusetts, 1976) and John A. Pitts, "The Association of Medical Superintendents of American Institutions for the Insane, 1844–1892: A Case Study of Specialism in American Medicine," (Ph.D. dissertation, University of Pennsylvania, 1979).

9. Most investigations of nineteenth-century psychiatry, such as Gerald Grob, *Mental Institutions in America: Social Policy to 1875* (New York: The Free Press, 1973) or Andrew Scull, *Museums of Madness: The Social Organization of Insanity in Nineteenth-Century England* (London: Allen Lane, 1979), are macroscopic studies which accord little attention to the social relationships within individual institutions. In contrast, see Tomes, *A Generous Confidence;* Peter L. Tyor and J. S. Zainaldin, "Asylum and Society: An Approach to Institutional Change," *Journal of Social History* 13, no. 1 (1979): 23–48; J. K. Walton, "Lunacy in the Industrial Revolution: A Study of Asylum Admissions in Lancashire, 1848–1850," *Journal of Social History* 13, no. 1 (1979): 1–22. The issue is discussed in general terms in Bill Luckin, "Towards a Social History of Institutionalization," *Social History* 8, no. 1 (1983): 87–94.

10. Traditional medical historiography suggests that psychiatric thought "reflected" social theory, thereby implying two explicitly separate categories of thought. See Norman Dain, *Concepts of Insanity in the United States, 1789–1865* (New Brunswick, N.J.: Rutgers University Press, 1964), p. *xiv* and Vieda Skultans, *English Madness: Ideas on Insanity, 1580–1890* (London: Routledge and Kegan Paul, 1979), p. 140. A number of recent studies, however, have argued convincingly that medical knowledge and social theory are inextricably enmeshed such that neither category is an epiphenomenon of the other. See Peter Wright and Andrew Treacher, eds., *The Problem of Medical Knowledge: Examin-*

ing the *Social Construction of Medicine* (Edinburgh: University of Edinburgh Press, 1982); Barry Barnes and Steven Shapin, eds., *Natural Order, Historical Studies of Scientific Culture* (Beverly Hills, Calif.: Sage Publications, 1979); Donald A. Mackenzie, *Statistics in Britain, 1865–1930, The Social Construction of Scientific Knowledge* (Edinburgh: University of Edinburgh Press, 1981). It is by no means necessary to adopt a rigid social constructionist methodology in order to emphasize the artificiality of the distinction between medical and social theory. See Charles Rosenberg, "Florence Nightingale on Contagion: The Hospital as Moral Universe," in his edited collection *Healing and History: Essays for George Rosen* (New York: Science History Publications, 1979), p. 129. Rosen himself argued a similar case in "Political Order and Human Health in Jeffersonian Thought," *BHM* 26, no. 1 (1952): 32–44.

CHAPTER 1 *The topography of a Victorian medical life*

1. James H. Coyne, "Richard M. Bucke – A Sketch," *Proceedings and Transactions of the Royal Society of Canada* 2nd series 12 (1906): 160–1; RMBC, Edwin Seaborn, "Life of Richard Maurice Bucke," unpublished manuscript, vol. 1: 35.
2. Coyne, "Richard M. Bucke," 162; C. K. Clarke, "Obituary, Richard Maurice Bucke," *AJI* 57 (1902): 724.
3. R. M. Bucke, *Cosmic Consciousness: A Study in the Evolution of the Human Mind* (Secaucus, N.J.: Citadel Press, 1977 [1901]), pp. 6–7.
4. RMBC, R. M. Bucke, "An Episode in the Life of R.M.B.," typed copy of original bound in vol. 4, Edwin Seaborn, "Richard Maurice Bucke in 21 Volumes"; R. M. Bucke, "Events in the Early Life of a Canadian Author," *The Bury and Norwich Post and Suffolk Herald* 13 July 1900, p. 7.
5. Bucke, "Life of R.M.B."; R. M. Bucke, "Twenty-five Years Ago." *The Overland Monthly* 2d ser., vol. 1 (June 1883) bound in Seaborn, "Bucke in 21 Volumes"; R. M. Bucke, "The Discovery of the Comstock," *London Advertiser* 16 Dec. 1897, bound in Seaborn, "Bucke in 21 Volumes" (from which pagination is cited), pp. 552, 554. If the wholesome prospecting community recalled by Bucke existed in 1858, it had changed dramatically by 1875. In that year 8.6% of the women in the area referred to by Bucke were acknowledged prostitutes. See Marion Goldman, "Sex and Commerce on the Comstock Lode," *Nevada Historical Society Quarterly* 21, no. 2 (1978): 98–129.
6. RMBC, Diary (12 March 1863–7 Dec. 1864): 5 May 1863.
7. Seaborn, "Life of Richard Maurice Bucke," vol. 1: 44; Coyne, "Richard M. Bucke," 170.
8. Harvey Cushing, *The Life of Sir William Osler* (London: Oxford University Press, 1949 [1925]), p. 71.
9. Stanley B. Frost, *McGill University for the Advancement of Learning,* vol. 1 (Montreal: McGill-Queen's University Press, 1980), ch. 6; Francis J. Shepherd, "The First Medical School in Canada, Its History and Founders, with Some Personal Reminiscences," *Canadian Medical Association Journal* 15 (April 1925): 420–1; Maurice Ewing, "The Influence of the Edinburgh Medical School in the Early Development of McGill University," *Canadian Journal of Surgery* 18 (May 1975): 287–96.
10. MUA, annual announcement of the Faculty of Medicine, "Faculty of Medicine of the University of McGill College, Montreal, 1859–60."
11. Shepherd, "First Medical School in Canada," 422.
12. Francis J. Shepherd, *Reminiscences of Student Days and Dissecting Room* (Montreal: privately printed, 1919), pp. 11, 19–20; idem, "First Medical School in Canada," 421; Sir William Osler, "An Address on the Medical Clinic: A Retrospect and a Forecast," *British Medical Journal* 1 (3 Jan. 1914): 10.
13. H. E. MacDermot, *A History of the Montreal General Hospital* (Montreal: Montreal General Hospital, 1950), pp. 52–3, 43–4; Shepherd, *Reminiscences of Student Days,* 16, 20–1.

166   Notes to pp. 9–11

14. Robert Craik, "Valedictory Address to the Graduates in Medicine of the University of McGill College, Montreal, 1863," in *Papers and Addresses* (Montreal: Gazette Printing Co., 1907), pp. 32–5; D. C. MacCallum, "Address, Introductory to the Course of Lectures on Medicine, Delivered to the Medical Class of McGill University, at the Opening of the Côté Street Building, November Fifth, Eighteen Hundred and Sixty," in *Addresses* (Montreal: Desbarats, 1901), pp. 77–82.
15. McGill University Archives: Faculty of Medicine; Shepherd, "First Medical School in Canada," 422.
16. Shepherd, "First Medical School in Canada," 2–5, 9–10; D. G. McCallum, "Sketches of Members of the McGill Medical Faculty, 1847–50," *McGill University Magazine* 3, no. 2 (1904): 166–8. Whatever its failings, it is doubtful that the standard or content of preclinical training at McGill differed significantly from leading British or American schools. See Gerald Geison, "Social and Institutional Factors in the Stagnancy of English Physiology, 1840–1870," *BHM* 45, no. 1 (1973): 39–47; S. T. Anning, "Provincial Medical Schools in the Nineteenth Century," in *The Evolution of Medical Education in Britain*, ed. F. N. L. Poynter (London: Pitman Medical, 1966), pp. 121–34; Jeanne Peterson, *The Medical Profession in Mid-Victorian London* (Berkeley, Calif.: University of California Press, 1978), pp. 56–8, 61–4; Martin Kaufman, *American Medical Education: The Formative Years, 1765–1910* (Westport, Conn.: Greenwood Press, 1976), ch. 6 and ch. 7; idem, *The University of Vermont College of Medicine* (Hanover, N.H.: University of Vermont College of Medicine/University Press of New England, 1979), ch. 5 and ch. 9; William Rothstein, *American Physicians in the Nineteenth Century* (Baltimore, Md.: Johns Hopkins University Press, 1972), ch. 15; Ronald L. Numbers, ed., *The Education of American Physicians: Historical Essays* (Berkeley, Calif.: University of California Press, 1980).
17. Shepherd, *Reminiscences of Student Days*, 12–13; Sir William Osler, "The Student Life," in *Aequanimitas*, 3rd ed. (New York: McGraw-Hill, n.d. [1905], pp. 420–1; "Obituary, Robert Palmer Howard," *Medical News* (Philadelphia) 54 (13 April 1889): 419. See also Maude Abbot, "Andrew F. Holmes, M.D., LL.D., 1797–1860," *McGill University Magazine* 4, no. 2 (1905): 176–81.
18. RMBC, R. M. Bucke, "Notes on Clinical Medicine and Surgery by Drs. McCallum [sic] and Craik, McGill College, 1861–1862"; D. C. MacCallum, "Address delivered to the Students of the Class of Clinical Medicine of McGill University, Session 1864–1865," in his *Addresses*, 163–4, 166–7. The general context in which such an approach developed is described in K. D. Keel, "Clinical Medicine," in *Medicine and Science in the 1860s*, ed. F. N. L. Poynter (London: Wellcome Institute for the History of Medicine, 1968), pp. 1–11. A perceptive commentary on this phase of American medicine is Edward C. Atwater, "Internal Medicine," in Numbers, *Education of American Physicians*, 143–74.
19. Peterson, *Medical Profession in Mid-Victorian London*, 65–7; F. F. Cartwright, "King's College Hospital," *History of Medicine* 4 (1972): 11–15.
20. John Woodward, *To Do the Sick No Harm: A Study of the British Voluntary Hospital System to 1875* (London: Routledge and Kegan Paul, 1974), pp. 34, 78; F. F. Cartwright, *A Social History of Medicine* (New York: Longman, 1977), p. 156; B. W. Thomas, "A Short Account of King's College Hospital," *Physiotherapy* 44 (10 May 1958): 130; W. E. Merrington, *University College Hospital and Its Medical School: A History* (London: Heineman, 1976), ch. 9; S. F. Holloway, "The All Saints' Sisterhood at University College Hospital, 1862–1899," *MH* 3, no. 2 (1959): 146–56; H. W. Lyle, *King's and Some King's Men* (Oxford: At the University Press, 1935), ch. 3.
21. Diary (12 March 1863–7 Dec. 1864): 12 March 1863; D. W. Taylor, "The Life and Teaching of William Sharpey (1802–1880), 'Father of Modern Physiology' in Britain," *MH* 15, no. 2 (1971): 126–53, and 15, no. 3 (1971): 241–59; J. C. Brougher, "William Sharpey (1802–1880)," *Annals of Medical History* 9, no. 2 (1972): 124–8.

22. Maurice Ewing, "Sir William Ferguson (1808–1877)," *Journal of the Royal College of Surgeons of Edinburgh* 22, no. 2 (1977): 127–35; J. P. Bennett, "Sir William Ferguson, Bart., 1808–1877," *Annals of the Royal College of Surgeons of England* 59 (1977): 484–6; Sir Gordon Gordon-Taylor, "Sir William Ferguson, Bt., F.R.C.S., F.R.S. (1808–1877)," *MH* 5, no. 1 (1961): 1–14; Diary (12 March 1863–7 Dec. 1864): 17 Oct. 1863.
23. Seaborn, "Life of Richard Maurice Bucke," vol. 1: 103; *Dictionary of National Biography* 16: 533–4; W. B. Ober, "Sir Henry Thompson, M.D. (1820–1904), Victorian Virtues," *New York State Journal of Medicine* 68, no. 19 (1968): 2571–7; R. K. Moxon, "Sir Henry Thompson (1820–1904)–Cremationist, Artist, and Host Extraordinary," *New England Journal of Medicine* 267, no. 18 (1 Nov. 1962): 927–9; Sir Zachary Cope, *The Versatile Victorian, Being the Life of Sir Henry Thompson, Bt., 1820–1904* (London: Harvey and Blythe, 1951), ch. 4 and ch. 5.
24. "Obituary," *Lancet* 2 (17 Dec. 1898): 1674–6; "Sir William Jenner (1815–1898)," *Journal of the American Medical Association* 214, no. 5 (2 Nov. 1970): 907–8; Seaborn, "Life of Richard Maurice Bucke," vol. 1: 103; RMBC, Biggs Andrews to Bucke, 4 Aug. 1872, and Bucke to H. B. Forman, 12 Dec. 1875.
25. Diary (12 March 1863–7 Dec. 1864): 3 Oct., 19 March 1863; Sir A. M. H. Gray, "Dermatologists at University College Hospital," *British Journal of Dermatology* 75 (Dec. 1963): 460–1; *Dictionary of National Biography* 16: 1938; Merrington, *University College Hospital*, 87–9; "A Brief Sketch of the Life of Sir John Russell Reynolds" in J. Russell Reynolds, *Essays and Addresses* (London: Macmillan, 1896), pp. *vii–xxi*; RMBC, Bucke to H. B. Forman, 19 Feb. 1869, 8 Nov. 1871, 11 May 1875, 24 Oct. 1877.
26. Maurice Ewing, "Jonathan Hutchinson, F.R.C.S.," *Annals of the Royal College of Surgeons of England* 57 (1975): 301. The scope of Hutchinson's interests is described in Herbert Hutchinson, *Jonathon Hutchinson, Life and Letters* (London: William Heinemann, 1946).
27. Diary (12 March 1863–7 Dec. 1864): 4 Dec. 1863. Bucke refers simply to "Hutchinson on 'Hereditary Syphilis'," but it is likely *A Clinical Memoir on Certain Disease of Ear and Eye, Consequent on Inherited Syphillis* (London: J. Churchill, 1863).
28. A. E. Wales, "Sir Jonathan Hutchinson, 1828–1913," *British Journal of Veneral Diseases* 39 (1963): 71–3; S. H. Greenblatt, "The Major Influences on the Early Life and Work of John Hughlings Jackson," *BHM* 39, no. 4 (1965): 354–6; Sir Jonathan Hutchinson, "Recollections of a Lifelong Friendship," in J. Hughlings Jackson, *Neurological Fragments* (London: Oxford University Press, n.d.), p. 37.
29. J. D. Rolleston, "Sir Benjamin Ward Richardson: His Life and Work," *Janus* 36 (1932): 361–83; Sir A. S. MacNalty, "The Work of Benjamin Ward Richardson: Its Effect on Modern Health Practice," *The Royal Sanitary Institute Journal* 75, no. 3 (March 1955): 201–10; J. H. Cassedy, "Hygeia: A Mid-Victorian Dream of a City of Health," *JHMAS* 17, no. 2 (April 1962): 217–28. On Beard see Charles Rosenberg, "The Place of George M. Beard in Nineteenth-Century Psychiatry," *BHM* 36, no. 3 (1962): 245–59.
30. RMBC, H. B. Forman to Bucke, 28 Nov. 1871, 29 May and 12 Sept. 1875; Bucke to H. B. Forman, 6 Oct., 12 Dec. 1875; Bucke to Forman, 6 Oct. 1875, 2 Feb. 1876.
31. Diary (12 March 1863–7 Dec. 1864): 15 April, 16 April, 29 April, 11 May, 15 May, 20 May, 25 May, 3 June, 6 June 1863. On Beau see K. Weismann, "J. H. S. Beau and his description of transverse depressions on nails," *British Journal of Dermatology* 97 (1977): 571–2.
32. Russell M. Jones, "American Doctors in Paris, 1820–1861: A Statistical Profile," *JHMAS* 25, no. 2 (1970): 143–56; idem, "American Doctors and the Parisian Medical World, 1830–1840)," *BHM* 47, no. 1 (1973): 40–65, and 47, no. 2 (1973): 177–204. No comparable Canadian studies exist, but see the tabular data on a slightly earlier period presented in Barbara Tunis, "Medical

Education and Medical Licensing in Lower Canada: Demographic Factors, Conflict, and Social Change," *Histoire Sociale–Social History* 14, no. 27 (1981): 67–91.

33. T. N. Bonner, *American Doctors and German Universities* (Lincoln, Nebr.: University of Nebraska Press, 1963), p. 23. An analysis of the 1,531 notable physicians listed in H. A. Kelly and W. L. Burrage, eds., *Dictionary of American Medical Biography* (New York: Appleton, 1928), revealed that 14.8% of the graduates in the first decade of the nineteenth century went abroad to study, while in the final decade this figure had risen to 36.6%. See Robert P. Hudson, "Abraham Flexner in Perspective: American Medical Education, 1865–1919," *BHM* 56, no. 6 (Nov.–Dec. 1972): 545–61.

34. Erwin H. Ackerknecht, "Elisha Bartlett and the Philosophy of the Paris Clinical School," *BHM* 24, no. 1 (1950): 43–60, 50–51; idem, *Medicine at the Paris Hospital, 1794–1848* (Baltimore, Md.: Johns Hopkins Press, 1967), especially ch. 1 and ch. 11; idem, "Medical Education in Nineteenth Century France," *Journal of Medical Education* 32, no. 2 (1957): 148–9; Jones, "Parisian Medical World," 52, 56, 198, 201; A. P. Carvadias, "The Mid-Nineteenth Century Clinical School of Paris," *Proceedings of the Royal Society of Medicine* 45 (Feb. 1952): 306–10.

35. Ackerknecht, *Medicine at the Paris Hospital*, 11, 112–13, 132, 134; Carvadias, "Clinical School of Paris," 306; F. H. Garrison, *An Introduction to the History of Medicine*, 4th ed. (Philadelphia, Penn.: W. B. Saunders, 1929), p. 613; A. D. Wright, "Two Great Surgeons," *History of Medicine* 2 (1975): 11–13; Jones, "Parisian Medical World," 177; Francis Schiller, *Paul Broca, Founder of French Anthropology, Explorer of the Brain* (Berkeley, Calif.: University of California Press, 1979), pp. 199–200.

36. Diary (12 March 1863–7 Dec. 1864): 12 June, 9 July, 17 July, 6 Aug., 26 March, 24 Dec., 10 Jan., 24 Jan. 1864. Bucke's other brother who became a physician, Augustus, died in India in 1857, as did two sisters, Alice and Anne, both of whom were married to British officers. George, the eldest brother, became a farmer; a brother Julian died at birth; and a sister, Helen, died in 1856. The two siblings to whom Bucke was closest were Philip ("Duke")–who was born in 1831 and worked for the postal service–and Julius, born in 1840, who later became a lawyer. This information is taken from the RMBC notebook entitled "Bucke Dates" by Edwin Seaborn and idem, "Life of Richard Maurice Bucke," vol. 1: 42, 49, 50.

37. Diary (12 March 1863–7 Dec. 1864): 5 March 1864, 4 Dec. 1863; RMBC, A. B. Grosh to Bucke, 22 Nov. 1863. The possibility of litigation was first mentioned in a letter from Grosh to Bucke, 27 April 1860. On the Comstock case and the general chaos of litigation arising from the mining claims in California and Nevada in the 1850s and 1860s, see Grant Smith, "The History of the Comstock Lode," *University of Nevada Bulletin* 37, no. 3, Geology and Mining Series (1943).

38. RMBC, Bucke to Jessie Gurd, 9 Nov. 1859 and 19 Aug. 1860; Diary (8 Dec. 1864–19 Oct. 1868): 22 July, 7 Sept., 23 Sept. 1865.

39. Elizabeth Macnab, *A Legal History of Health Professions in Ontario: A Study for the Committee on the Healing Arts* (Toronto: Queen's Printer, 1970), pp. 9–14. Background to this legislation is found in William Caniff, *The Medical Profession in Upper Canada, 1783–1850* (Toronto: William Briggs, 1894), Part II.

40. G. W. Spragge, "The Trinity Medical College," *Ontario History* 58, no. 2 (1966): 71–8; J. J. Heagerty, *Four Centuries of Medical History in Canada*, 2 vol. (Toronto: Macmillan, 1928), vol. 2, p. 121. Joseph F. Kett, "American and Canadian Medical Institutions, 1800–1870," in *Medicine in Canadian Society: Historical Perspectives* ed. S. E. D. Shortt (Montreal: McGill-Queen's University Press, 1981), pp. 189–205; M. A. Patterson, "The Life and Times of the Hon. John Rolph, M.D. (1793–1870)," *MH* 5, no. 1 (1961): 15–33.

41. H. E. MacDermot, *One Hundred Years of Medicine in Canada, 1867–1967* (Toronto: McClelland and Stewart, 1967), pp. 152–5; C. G. Roland, "Ontario

Medical Periodicals as Mirrors of Change," *Ontario History* 72, no. 1 (1980): 3–15; idem, and P. Potter, *An Annotated Bibliography of Canadian Medical Periodicals, 1826–1975* (Toronto: Hannah Institute for the History of Medicine, 1979), pp. 64–5.

42. In its essential features, the professionalization of Canadian medicine differed little from the process as it occurred in the United States and Great Britain. See S. E. D. Shortt, "Physicians, Science, and Status: Issues in the Professionalization of Medicine in the Nineteenth Century," *MH* 27, no. 1 (1983): 51–68; Peterson, *Medical Profession in Mid-Victorian London;* Noel Parry and Jose Parry, *The Rise of the Medical Profession: A Study of Collective Social Mobility* (London: Croom Helm, 1976), pp. 104–61; Joseph F. Kett, *The Formation of the American Medical Profession: The Roles of Institutions, 1780–1860* (Westport, Conn.: Greenwood Press, 1980 [1968]); Rothstein, *American Physicians;* Paul Starr, *The Social Transformation of American Medicine* (New York: Basic Books, 1982).

43. Midcentury general practice was a strange blend of professional growth and therapeutic stagnation. See Ivan Waddington, "General Practitioners and Consultants in Early Nineteenth-Century England: The Sociology of an Intra-Professional Conflict," in *Health Care and Popular Medicine in Nineteenth Century England: Essays in the Social History of Medicine,* eds. John Woodward and David Richards (London: Croom Helm, 1977), pp. 166–88; Charles Rosenberg, "The Practice of Medicine in New York a Century Ago," *BHM* 41, no. 3 (1967): 223–58.

44. W. G. Crosbie, *The Toronto General Hospital, 1819–1965: A Chronicle* (Toronto: Macmillan, 1975), pp. 57, 71; Abraham Groves, *All in the Day's Work: Leaves from a Doctor's Casebook* (Toronto: Macmillan, 1934), p. 3. See also C. G. Roland, "The Early Years of Antiseptic Surgery in Canada," in Shortt, *Medicine in Canadian Society,* pp. 237–53.

45. Charles Rosenberg, "The Therapeutic Revolution: Medicine, Meaning, and Social Change in Nineteenth-Century America," in *The Therapeutic Revolution: Essays in the Social History of American Medicine,* eds. Charles Rosenberg and Morris Vogel (Philadelphia, Penn.: University of Pennsylvania Press, 1979), pp. 3–25; MacDermot, *Medicine in Canada,* p. 22; Heagerty, *Medical History in Canada,* 2: 90–3. On malaria in Midwestern North America see Erwin Ackerknecht, *Malaria in the Upper Mississippi Valley* (Baltimore Md.: Johns Hopkins Press, 1945). For an informative description of midcentury pharmaceuticals, see John S. Haller, *American Medicine in Transition, 1840–1910* (Chicago: University of Chicago Press, 1981), ch. 3.

46. Geoffrey Bilson, *A Darkened House: Cholera in Nineteenth Century Canada* (Toronto: University of Toronto Press, 1980); Heagerty, *Medical History in Canada,* vol. 2: Part 1; Katherine McCuaig, " 'From Social Reform to Social Service.' The Changing Role of Volunteers: the Anti-tuberculosis Campaign, 1900–1930." *Canadian Historial Review* 61, no. 4 (1980): 480–501; George J. Wherrett, *The Miracle of the Empty Beds: A History of Tuberculosis in Canada* (Toronto: University of Toronto Press, 1977), ch. 1.

47. On transportation in general practice for a somewhat later period, see S. E. D. Shortt, "The Family Doctor in Canada, 1900–1950," *Canadian Family Physician* 22 (June 1976): 58; M. L. Berger, "The Influence of the Automobile on Rural Health Care, 1900–1929," *JHMAS* 28, no. 4 (1973): 319–35.

48. The literature on medical fee collection in Canada is scant and 70% is an estimate. See Charles Godfrey, *Medicine for Ontario: A History* (Belleville, Ontario: Mika Publishing, 1979), pp. 202–4; Shortt, "Family Doctor in Canada," 58–9; Dan McCaughey, "The Overcrowding of the Medical Profession in Ontario: 1851–1911," paper presented at the Annual Meeting of the American Association for the History of Medicine, Toronto, May 1981; K. F. Clute, *The General Practitioner: A Study of Medical Education and Practice in Ontario and Nova Scotia* (Toronto: University of Toronto Press, 1963), pp. 175–212. More generally, see George Rosen, *Fees and Fee Bills, Some Economic Aspects of Medical*

Practice in Nineteenth-Century America (Baltimore, Md.: Johns Hopkins Press, 1947).
49. Clute, General Practitioner, 246. See also J. H. Barber et al., General Practice Medicine (Edinburgh: Churchill Livingstone, 1973), p. 5; John Fry et al., Scientific Foundations of Family Medicine (Chicago: Year Medical Publishers, 1978), p. 5.
50. I. Greenwald, "The History of Goitre in Canada," Canadian Medical Association Journal 84 (Feb. 1961): 379–88, documents that thyroid deficiency was quite common in nineteenth-century Ontario. James Harvey Young suggests that the "widespread biliousness" in the "dietary dark ages" of nineteenth-century America derived from the "national habit" of overeating. See his The Medical Messiahs: A Social History of Health Quackery in Twentieth-Century America (Princeton, N.J.: Princeton University Press, 1967), p. 20.
51. RMBC, Sarnia Casebook Number 2, 27 June 1867–16 Aug. 1896; Diary (8 Dec. 1864–19 Oct. 1868): 15 Oct., 2 Nov. 1865, 14 Jan., 17 Jan. 1866. On calomel, a mercury purgative, see Haller, American Medicine in Transition, 77–90.
52. Diary (8 Dec. 1864–19 Oct. 1868): 18 July, 19 July, 9 Aug., 17 Oct., 30 Dec. 1865. Bucke to H. B. Forman, 3 Dec. 1869 (continuation of a letter dated 29 Oct. 1869).
53. William Victor Johnson described an almost identical caseload in the 1920s and 1930s in an area 120 miles northeast of Sarnia. See his Before the Age of Miracles: Memoirs of a Country Doctor (Toronto: Fitzhenry and Whiteside, 1975), p. 4.
54. RMBC, Medical Ledger A, Sarnia, 26 Sept. 1865–10 July 1871; Bucke to H. B. Forman, 11 April 1869, 1 Dec. 1869 (continuation of a letter dated 29 Oct. 1869), 11 April 1870.
55. RMBC, Bucke to H. B. Forman, 24 Nov. 1868, 11 April 1869, 29 Oct. 1869; Edwin Seaborn, notebook entitled, "Bucke Dates." Bucke's Medical Ledger C, Sarnia, 18 March 1869–10 Aug. 1870, suggests his average fee per consultation was $1.25.
56. RMBC, Alfred Forman to Bucke, 24 Oct. 1879; Diary (8 Dec. 1864–19 Oct. 1868): 26 Feb. 1866, 4 March 1866, 19 Oct. 1868.
57. RMBC, Bucke to H. B. Forman, 2 Oct. 1870, 11 Sept. 1871, 7 Dec. 1871; Biggs Andrews to Bucke, 4 Aug. 1872.
58. RMBC, Diary (12 March 1863–7 Dec. 1864): 12 March 1863, 11 Sept. 1864; Biggs Andrews to Bucke, 26 Sept. 1876; Diary (1 Jan. 1878–19 Nov. 1878); 30 July 1878. For a contemporary clinical description of acute anxiety or panic attacks very similar to Bucke's, see Kurt J. Isselbacher et al., Harrison's Principles of Internal Medicine, 9th ed. (New York: McGraw-Hill, 1980), p. 70, and D. V. Sheehan, "Panic Attacks and Phobias," New England Journal of Medicine 307 (15 July 1982): 156–8. Rarely, psychomotor epilepsy might present in this fashion.
59. R. M. Bucke, "The Functions of the Great Sympathetic Nervous System," AJI 34 (Oct. 1877): 142–3; RMBC, Bucke to H. B. Forman, 4 July 1878.
60. William James, The Varieties of Religious Experience (New York: Collier Macmillan, 1979 [1902]), pp. 313–14.
61. Bucke, Cosmic Consciousness, 8.
62. RMBC, Bucke to H. B. Forman, 10 Dec. 1872.
63. RMBC, Diary (8 Dec. 1864–19 Oct. 1868): 30 Nov. 1865, 19 Jan., 24 Jan. 1866; Bucke to H. B. Forman, 3 Oct. 1873, 3 Nov. 1873.
64. RMBC, Bucke to Forman, 27 Dec. 1871, 8 Nov. 1871, 17 July 1872.
65. RMBC, Bucke to H. B. Forman, 30 Sept. 1873, 22 July 1874; J. T. Saywell, "The Early History of Canadian Oil Companies: A Chapter in Canadian Business History," Ontario History 53, no. 1 (1961): 67–8; Victor Ross, Petroleum in Canada (n.p., 1917), p. 18; Jean Elford and Edward Phelps, "Oil, Then and Now," Canadian Geographical Journal 77, no. 5 (1968): 168–9.
66. RMBC, Bucke to H. B. Forman, 6 Oct. 1875.
67. RMBC, Bucke to H. B. Forman, 12 Dec. 1875, 2 Feb. 1876.

CHAPTER 2 *The human ecology of the London Asylum*

1. T. E. Brown, " 'Living with God's Afflicted': A History of the Provincial Lunatic Asylum at Toronto, 1830–1911" (Ph.D. dissertation, Queen's University, 1980), pp. 195–8.
2. ARMS (1881): 353. On Rockwood, see Catherine Sims, "An Institutional History of the Asylum for the Insane at Kingston, 1856–1885," (M.A. essay, Queen's University, 1981).
3. Calculated from figures in Richard Splane, *Social Welfare in Ontario, 1791–1893* (Toronto: University of Toronto Press, 1965), pp. 282–3, 63.
4. ARMS (1877): 273, (1878): 308.
5. IR (1879): 32–3.
6. ARMS (1883): 84. As late as 1898, the asylum's annual budget exceeded that of the city of London. *London* (Ontario) *Free Press* 10 June 1898.
7. IR (1881): 34.
8. ARMS (1877): 274; IR (1881): 29; ARMS (1886): 23.
9. ARMS (1877): 279.
10. IR (1887): 34.
11. ARMS (1881): 351; IR (1883): 55.
12. ARMS (1885): 68, (1884): 84. The London Asylum was hardly unique in its structural deficiencies. See, for example, T. E. Brown's description of the Toronto Asylum in " 'Architecture as Therapy'," *Archivaria* 10 (Summer 1980): 117–23. Nor were these faults confined to Canada. See W. H. Parry-Jones, *The Trade in Lunacy* (London: Routledge and Kegan Paul, 1972), pp. 249–59.
13. D. H. Tuke, *The Insane in the United States and Canada* (London: H. K. Lewis, 1885), pp. 219–20.
14. ARMS (1881): 352; IR (1879): 32, (1881): 34.
15. IR (1881): 30.
16. RMBC, Bucke to H. B. Forman, 6 Oct. 1875.
17. RMBC, Bucke to H. B. Forman, 2 Feb. 1876. See also the similar letter of 18 March 1877.
18. RMBC, Bucke to H. B. Forman, 6 Dec. 1881.
19. RMBC, Bucke to H. B. Forman, 8 July 1879.
20. RMBC, Bucke to H. B. Forman, 5 June 1882.
21. RMBC, Bucke to H. B. Forman, 22 May 1881. Bucke informed Forman that he had "been given the job of organizing the Medical Faculty . . . I shall probably take a chair myself." In fact, Bucke seems to have been simply one of a group who organized to form the school. See J. J. Talman and R. D. Talman, *"Western"–1878–1953* (London, Ontario: University of Western Ontario, 1953), pp. 30–3. A similar though briefer account is found in Murray L. Barr, *A Century of Medicine in Western* (London, Ontario: University of Western Ontario, 1977), pp. 76–8.
22. The Inspector had opposed Bucke's initial academic appointment. IC: vol. 223: S. C. Wood to Inspector, 13 Sept. 1881. The opposition to his appointment as Dean is detailed in IC: vol. 231: R. M. Bucke to W. T. O'Reilly, 30 August 1886, and W. T. O'Reilly to Bucke, 1 Sept. 1886.
23. RMBC, Bucke to H. B. Forman, 8 July 1879 and 6 Dec. 1881.
24. RMBC, Bucke to H. B. Forman, 26 Nov. 1876.
25. RMBC, Diary (1 Jan. 1878–19 Nov. 1878): passim.
26. RMBC, Bucke to H. B. Forman, 26 Nov. 1876.
27. ARMS (1879): 331.
28. University of Western Ontario, D. B. Weldon Library: Diary of Dr. Charles Sippi, 1893–1897, Addenda by Emilio Goggio, "The Italian Contribution to the Development of Music in Ontario."
29. Sippi Diary: 25 Dec. 1893, 1 Aug. 1896, 18 May 1893.
30. IC: vol. 229: J. W. Langmuir to the Provincial Secretary, 9 Jan. 1877; Langmuir

to Dr. Stephen Lett, 9 Jan. 1877; Bucke to Langmuir, 30 Aug. 1877; Bucke to Langmuir, 29 March 1877; Langmuir to Lett, 25 April 1877.

31. IC: vol. 218: Bucke to Robert Christie, 29 March 1895; ibid.: vol. 221: 20 June 1898: "Investigation at North Building in re. Dr. Buchan vs. Mrs. Martin. Conducted by Inspector Christie."

32. IC: vol. 231: W. T. O'Reilly to A. S. Hardy, 25 July 1887; O'Reilly to Bucke, 23 Aug. 1887.

33. ARMS (1898): 75.

34. See, for example: IC: vol. 227: Bucke to Robert Christie, 21 Sept. 1901, complaining that an assistant had typhoid fever.

35. IC: vol. 218: "Numbers of Officers and Employees with salaries for 1889." The three assistants earned $1100, $900, and $800, respectively. In private practice, an income of $2000 was a not-unreasonable expectation. See J. R. Clouston, "The Country Practitioner of Today," *Montreal Medical Journal* (31 Oct. 1902): 780. On Pensions, see IC: vol. 220: Provincial Secretary to A. T. Hobbs, 12 April 1901.

36. IC: vol. 227: T. Millman to J. W. Langmuir, 16 Feb. 1881; Bucke to Langmuir, 16 Feb. 1881; Langmuir to Bucke, 19 Feb. 1881.

37. See, for example, the transfers reported in ARMS (1895): 39.

38. ARMS (1883): 84.

39. IMB (2 Jan. 1879): 17.

40. MSJ, 14 Feb. 1877–31 Aug. 1884. A typical entry indicative of brief patient contact is that of 14 Feb. 1879: "Went through all the halls–saw all the patients."

41. IC: vol. 17: Bucke to J. W. Langmuir, 9 July 1881; ibid.: vol. 221: Robert Christie to Bucke, 15 Nov. 1895; Bucke to Christie, 16 Nov. 1895.

42. IR (1883): 53.

43. LC, Feinberg Whitman Collection: Bucke to Walt Whitman, 27 Aug. 1888.

44. IMB (15 Jan. 1884): 208. See, for example: R. M. Bucke, "A Short History of Sewage Disposal at the Asylum for the Insane, London, Ontario," *Canadian Engineer* 6 (Oct. 1898): 155–6.

45. Bonnie E. Blustein, " 'A Hollow Square of Psychological Science': American Neurologists and Psychiatrists in Conflict," in *Madhouses, Mad-Doctors, and Madmen: The Social History of Psychiatry in the Victorian Era* ed. A. T. Scull (Philadelphia, Penn.: University of Pennsylvania Press, 1981), pp. 241–70; David Rothman, *Conscience and Convenience: The Asylum and Its Alternatives In Progressive America* (Boston, Mass.: Little, Brown, 1980), ch. 9.

46. RMBC, Bucke to H. Traubel, 26 July 1890.

47. RMBC, Bucke to H. Traubel, 1 March 1892.

48. IC: vol. 218: "Salaries and Perquisites of Asylum Superintendents," 1895, 1896. See above, note 17.

49. IR (1894): *xiv*.

50. IR (1892): 42. Sippi Diary: 12 April 1894, 27 January 1897.

51. ARMS (1894): 34. Bucke requested to no avail that his house be painted in his reports from 1891 to 1894. The apparent economizing in the early 1890s during recession years may have been sparked by the antimedical and anti-institutional aspects of contemporary agrarian protest. See S. E. D. Shortt, "Social Change and Political Crisis in Rural Ontario: The Patrons of Industry, 1889–1896," in *Oliver Mowat's Ontario,* ed. Donald Swainson (Toronto: Macmillan, 1972), pp. 211–35. The matter of leave was discussed between the Inspector and the Attorney General. See IC: vol. 231: J. W. Langmuir to A. S. Wood, 2 Feb. 1880; Wood to Langmuir, 6 Feb. 1880; Langmuir to Bucke, 20 Feb. 1880.

52. ARMS (1884): 70.

53. IC: vol. 232: Bucke to J. W. Langmuir, "Re American Asylums," n.d., RMBC, Diary (1 Jan. 1878–19 Nov. 1878): 19 Feb. and 13 Nov. 1878.

54. Resignation prior to retirement meant the loss of pension rights. See IC: vol. 220: Provincial Secretary to A. T. Hobbs, 12 April 1901. Leaving the asylum to

begin private practice during the 1880s and 1890s would have been economically difficult. See Daniel McCaughey, "The Overcrowding of the Profession: Ontario, 1870–1914," paper presented at the annual meeting of the American Association for the History of Medicine, Toronto, May 1981.

55. The best description of the Inspector's duties is that given by J. W. Langmuir in IR (1878): 1–3. See also Splane, *Social Welfare in Ontario*, 44–53. The Canadian context for Inspectorship legislation is sketched in J. E. Hodgetts, *Pioneer Public Service: An Administrative History of the United Canadas, 1841–1867* (Toronto: University of Toronto Press, 1955). On the inspection of British asylums see D. J. Mellett, "Bureaucracy and Mental Illness: The Commissioners of Lunacy, 1845–1890," *MH* 25, no. 3 (1981): 221–50.

56. RMBC, Bucke to Harry Forman, 10 Dec. 1872. Duke University, Perkins Library: Trent Collection: Bucke to Walt Whitman, 18 Jan. 1889.

57. See O'Reilly's appraisal of Bucke's work in IR (1887): 36. For Christie, in contrast, see above, note 41, on the dispute over appropriate selections for the patient library. Christie was skeptical about Bucke's gynecological surgery. See Sippi Diary: 8 Oct. 1897.

58. G. M. Rose, ed., *A Cyclopedia of Canadian Biography* (Toronto: Rose Publishing, 1886), pp. 64–5. See also Stephen Connors, "J. W. Langmuir and the Development of Prisons and Reformatories in Ontario, 1868–1882" (M.A. thesis, Queen's University, 1982), and Splane, *Social Welfare in Ontario*, 44–51.

59. Sippi Diary: 8 Oct. 1897. Feinberg Whitman Collection: Bucke to Walt Whitman, 11 Oct. 1888.

60. RMBC, Bucke to Horace Traubel, 2 Dec. 1890.

61. IR (1883): 55.

62. RMBC, Bucke to Horace Traubel, 7 Oct. 1888.

63. See, for example: IR (1881): 33.

64. See above, note 31.

65. IR (1878): 36, (1879): 34, (1883): 53, (1881): 29, 32.

66. IMB 25–6 (Nov. 1879): 62. Such concerns were not unique to Ontario. See Peter McCandless, " 'Build! Build!' The Controversy over the Case of the Chronically Insane in England, 1855–1870," *BHM* 53, no. 4 (1979): 553–74.

67. IR (1892): 1–2.

68. IMB 25–6 (Nov. 1879): 63.

69. The proportion of certificates to warrant admissions in Ontario asylums seems to have remained relatively stable. Between 1871 and 1896, the latter exceeded the former in 1874, 1876, and 1886. IR (1896): xiii.

70. IR (1884): 38.

71. IR (1896): xiii. M. C. Urquhart and K. C. Buckley, *Historical Statistics of Canada* (New York: Cambridge University Press, 1965), p. 14. The crowding of the London Asylum experience was by no means an exception. See Brown, "Living with God's Afflicted," 133–9, for the Toronto Asylum and for Kingston see Sims, "Asylum for the Insane at Kingston," ch. 2. A similar phenomenon was noted in the United States. See Gerald N. Grob, *Mental Institutions in America: Social Policy to 1875* (New York: Free Press, 1973), pp. 307–8. Similarly, British institutions were filled to the limit. See A. T. Scull, *Museums of Madness: The Social Organization of Insanity in Nineteenth-Century England* (London: Allen Lane, 1979), pp. 186–98.

72. IMB (10 July 1879): 55.

73. Splane, *Social Welfare in Ontario*, 282–3; IR (1879): 24, (1894): 18.

74. See, for example, IR (1887): 19. The cost of medical supplies that year was $0.82 per patient, while total cost of maintenance was $134.40.

75. IMB (2 Jan. 1879): 17; IR (1879): 36.

76. IMB (27 March 1879): 39.

77. IR (1886): 32–3, (1887): 2, 29. IC: vol. 67: Robert Christie to Manager, Toronto General Trust Company, 26 Oct. 1893.

78. Urquhart and Buckley, *Historical Statistics of Canada*, 291, 94–5.

79. See above, note 3.
80. IC: vol. 230: R. Mathison to J. W. Langmuir, 19 Feb. 1877.
81. IC: vol. 231: C. J. Colwell to W. T. O'Reilly, 15 July 1889. Note also vol. 73: Anonymous to Robert Christie, 28 Feb. 1902.
82. *London (Ontario) Free Press* 10 June 1898.
83. Sippi Diary: 16 Oct. 1897. American Asylum positions were certainly awarded for political reasons. See Grob, *Mental Institutions in America*, 213.
84. IC: vol. 227: Robert Christie to Bucke, 2 Oct. 1896.
85. IC: vol. 218: T. S. Hobbs to Robert Christie, 14 Jan. 1897. On Hobbs, see *The Canadian Who's Who* (London: The Times, 1910), p. 107.
86. IC: vol. 224: Robert Christie to the Provincial Treasurer, 7 April 1898.
87. The same was true of the English asylum service. See Richard Hunter and Ida Macalpine, *Psychiatry for the Poor: 1851 Colney Hatch Asylum, Friern Hospital, 1973: A Medical and Social History* (London: Dawsons, 1974), p. 17.
88. Quoted in Rothman, *Conscience and Convenience*, 296. While asylums became less medical and more bureaucratic, general hospitals were in the process of displacing lay values with medical authority. See Charles Rosenberg, "Inward Vision and Outward Glance: The Shaping of the American Hospital, 1880–1914," *BHM* 53, no. 3 (1979): 346–91.
89. Similar principles are noted in the evolution of late nineteenth-century factories. See Daniel Nelson, *Managers and Workers: Origins of the New Factory System in the United States, 1880–1920* (Madison, Wis.: University of Wisconsin Press, 1975), pp. ix, 57, 59.
90. Splane, *Social Welfare in Ontario*, 50.
91. See Samuel Haber, *Efficiency and Uplift: Scientific Management in the Progressive Era, 1890–1920* (Chicago: University of Chicago Press, 1964); Martin J. Schiesl, *The Politics of Efficiency: Municipal Administration and Reform in America, 1800–1920* (Berkeley, Calif.: University of California Press, 1977); Raymond E. Callahan, *Education and the Cult of Efficiency: A Study of the Social Forces that Have Shaped the Administration of Public Schools* (Chicago: University of Chicago Press, 1962). On the medical aspects of such beliefs, see George Rosen, "The Efficiency Criterion in Medical Care, 1900–1920: An Early Approach to an Evaluation of Health Service," *BHM* 50, no. 1 (1976): 28–46.
92. The prototype state welfare institutions of nineteenth-century Canada coexisted with voluntarism, a system whose scant concern for efficiency spelled its eventual demise. See Stephen Speisman, "Munificent Parsons and Municipal Parsimony: Voluntary vs. Public Poor Relief in Nineteenth-Century Toronto," *Ontario History* 65, no. 1 (1973): 32–49. See also Roy Lubove, *The Professional Altruist: The Emergence of Social Work as a Career, 1880–1930* (New York: Atheneum, 1980 [1965]), ch. 1.
93. For the United States, Great Britain, and Ireland, see Grob, *Mental Institutions in America*, 215; Scull, *Museums of Madness*, 122, 182; Mark Finane, *Insanity and the Insane in Post-Famine Ireland* (London: Croom Helm, 1981), p. 178.
94. Eric Carlson and Norman Dain, "The Psychotherapy that Was Moral Treatment," *American Journal of Psychiatry* 117 (Dec. 1960): 519–24; J. S. Bockoven, "Moral Treatment in American Psychiatry," *Journal of Nervous and Mental Diseases* 124 (Aug. 1956): 167–94; Alexander Walk, "Some Aspects of 'Moral Treatment' of the Insane up to 1850," *Journal of Mental Science* 100 (Oct. 1954): 807–37.
95. W. F. Bynum, "Rationales for Therapy in British Psychiatry: 1780–1835," *MH* 18, no. 4 (1974): 332–4; Scull, *Museums of Madness*, 132–41.
96. John Conolly, *The Construction and Government of Lunatic Asylums and Hospitals for the Insane* (London: Dawson, 1968 [1847]), p. 83.
97. Rosenberg, "Inward Vision and Outward Glance," 347.
98. Charles Rosenberg, "And Heal the Sick: The Hospital and the Patient in Nineteenth-Century America," *Journal of Social History* 10, no. 4 (1977): 428. Historians are showing an increased interest in the "inner world of the asylum."

Compare, for example, Gerald Grob's *The State and the Mentally Ill: A History of Worcester State Hospital in Massachusetts, 1830–1920* (Chapel Hill, N.C.: University of North Carolina Press, 1966), which focuses almost exclusively on policy makers and physicians, with John Walton's attempt to explore the asylum subculture in, "The Treatment of Pauper Lunatics in Victorian England: The Case of the Lancaster Asylum, 1816–1870," in Scull, *Madhouses, Mad-Doctors, and Madmen*, 166–97. See also Nancy Tomes, *A Generous Confidence: Thomas Story Kirkbride and the Art of Asylum-keeping, 1841–1883* (New York: Cambridge University Press, 1984), ch. 5.

99. Historical literature on asylum attendants is scant but see the following: Mick Carpenter, "Asylum Nursing Before 1914: A Chapter in the History of Labour," in *Rewriting Nursing History*, ed. Celia Davies (London: Croom Helm, 1980), pp. 123–46; F. R. Adams, "From Association to Union: Professional Organization of Asylum Attendants, 1869–1919," *British Journal of Sociology* 20, no. 1 (1969): 11–26; L. F. Stevens and D. D. Henrie, "A History of Psychiatric Nursing," *Bulletin of the Menninger Clinic* 30, no. 1 (1966): 32–8; Alexander Walk, "The History of Mental Nursing," *Journal of Mental Science* 107 (Jan. 1961): 1–17; Richard Hunter, "The Rise and Fall of Mental Nursing," *Lancet* (14 Jan. 1956): 98–9; E. H. Santos and E. Stainbrook, "A History of Psychiatric Nursing in the Nineteenth Century," *JHMAS* 4, no. 1 (1949): 48–74.

100. IR (1897): 23, (1887): 21, ARMS (1898): 71, (1888): 25.
101. ARMS (1886): 30.
102. Walk, "History of Mental Nursing," 8; ARMS (1892): 41.
103. Carpenter, "Asylum Nursing," 128; IC: vol. 221: Christie to Dr. McCallum, 13 Aug. 1902; Hunter, "Rise and Fall of Mental Nursing," 98.
104. Stevens and Henrie, "History of Psychiatric Nursing," 33.
105. ARMS (1879): 333; IC: vol. 228: Bucke to O'Reilly, 22 Feb. 1886.
106. RMBC, MSOB, IC: vol. 229: Bucke to W. T. O'Reilly, 27 Sept. 1886. A similar controversy occurred in the U.S. and Britain. See Santos and Stainbrook, "Psychiatric Nursing in the Nineteenth Century," 55, and Walk, "History of Mental Nursing," 13.
107. MSJ: 25 July 1878.
108. ARMS (1881): 352.
109. MSOB: 1 Nov. 1882.
110. Ibid.: 20 Nov. 1881.
111. Ibid.: 20 April 1880. The patients' diet is described in ARMS (1877): 275, and that of the attendants in IC: vol. 228: Bucke to J. W. Langmuir, 6 July 1881.
112. Carpenter, "Asylum Nursing," 130–2, describes a somewhat similar role among English attendants. Many were required to live in and most functioned as work supervisors and security enforcers.
113. AS (microfilm): vol. 1: 16, "At the Asylum, Annual Ball and Entertainment," n.d. (1877?).
114. AS: vol. 2: 129, "In the Asylum," 30 Dec. 1897.
115. AS: vol. 1: 3, "A Pleasant Night which Is Passed at the Asylum," n.d. (1879?).
116. A high turnover rate was common in the United States and Ireland. See Grob, *Mental Institutions in America*, 213, and Finnane, *Insanity and the Insane*, 179.
117. Anglo-American asylums were notorious for very low wages and long hours. On the United States, see Grob, *Mental Institutions in America*, 213, 215; Santos and Stainbrook, "Psychiatric Nursing in the Nineteenth Century," 57. On England and Ireland, see Hunter and Macalpine, *Psychiatry for the Poor*, 92–5; Carpenter, "Asylum Nursing," 131–2, 143; Adams, "From Association to Union," 15; Finnane, *Insanity and the Insane*, 179–81.
118. IC: vol. 221: Bucke to Robert Christie, 8 Feb. 1895; ibid.: vol. 228: Bucke to J. W. Langmuir, 6 July 1881.
119. IC: vol. 229: W. T. O'Reilly to Thomas Short, 29 April 1887.
120. ARMS (1882): 74; Urquhart and Buckley, *Historical Statistics of Canada*, 95.
121. ARMS (1881): 358.

122. IC: vol. 218: "Number of Officers and Employees with salaries for 1899"; Urquhart and Buckley, *Historical Statistics of Canada*, 94.
123. IC: vol. 218: Bucke to Robert Christie, 23 April 1895.
124. ARMS (1881): 358; IR (1879): 61, (1880): 68, (1881): 66.
125. IC: vol. 218: Bucke to Robert Christie, 23 April 1895. These figures include a mixture of discharges and resignations.
126. IC: vol. 229: Bucke to O'Reilly, 29 March 1886.
127. IC: vol. 228: Henry Landon to J. W. Langmuir, 11 June 1875.
128. ARMS (1877): 275.
129. Ontario Archives: RG10, 20-C-4, vol. 1: London Asylum, Register of Employees, 1870–1923, 1877. Hereafter cited as Register.
130. AS: vol. 1: 16, "At the Asylum, Annual Ball and Entertainment," n.d. (1877?).
131. IMB: 2 July 1881.
132. ARMS (1882): 72. IC: vol. 17: Bucke to J. W. Langmuir, 25 June 1881; ibid.: vol. 229: Bucke to Langmuir, 28 Nov. 1881. MSJ: 17 Sept. 1877, 9 Oct. 1879, 23 June 1887.
133. MSJ: 23 Oct. 1877, 27 July 1879. RMBC, Bucke to Horace Traubel, 22 Jan. 1891. IC: vol. 218: J. R. Cartwright to Robert Christie, 19 Oct. 1891; Bucke to Christie, 23 Aug. 1890.
134. MSJ: 7 and 8 April 1877; 7 Dec. 1877; 21 Feb. 1878; 1 July 1881.
135. MSJ: 26 June 1877; IC: vol. 224: Bucke to Robert Christie, 10 Sept. 1897.
136. Register, 1877, 1887, 1897. Dispensing discipline to attendants was an important function of British and Irish Superintendents. See Carpenter, "Asylum Nursing," 137; Adams, "From Association to Union," 17; Finnane, *Insanity and the Insane*, 177.
137. AS: vol. 2: 129, "In the Asylum," 30 Dec. 1897.
138. IC: vol. 17: Bucke to J. W. Langmuir, 31 July 1881.
139. IR (1878): 21.
140. MSJ: 15 Aug. 1881.
141. For the size of seventy major American asylums see Grob, *Mental Institutions in America,* appendix IV. Of these, a dozen exceeded the London Asylum population, while half a dozen were roughly equal to it. The London figures are taken from ARMS (1877) and yearly during the 1890s.
142. Gareth Stedman Jones, "Class Expression versus Social Control? A Critique of Recent Trends in the Social History of Leisure," *History Workshop* 4 (Autumn 1977): 163. For a contemporary attempt to capture the patient experience, see Michael Glenn, ed., *Voices from the Asylum* (New York: Harper and Row, 1974).
143. IC: vol. 229: R. Mathison to J. W. Langmuir, 2 April 1877; Langmuir to Mathison, 4 April 1877.
144. FCB: vol. 2: 16.
145. FCB: vol. 4: 136.
146. IR (1892): 1–2; (1896): xvii.
147. IR (1885): 29–30. See also Henry Landor's earlier but similar opinion, ARMS (1872): 156. In as many as 50% of admissions, the duration of illness was said to be less than three months (ARMS (1885): 82), suggesting possibly inaccurate information or very limited tolerance on the part of relatives or civic authorities. More likely is the probability that the onset of illness was assigned to the point at which a chronic disability became florid in its symptomatology, such that neither patient nor family could continue to cope adequately.
148. ARMS (1879): 348; (1890): 86.
149. On the ambiguous relationship between age and asylum incarceration see Barbara Rosenkrantz and Maris Vinovskis, "The Invisible Lunatics: Old Age and Insanity in Midnineteenth-Century Massachusetts," in *Aging and the Elderly,* eds. S. F. Spicker et al. (Atlantic Highlands, N.J.: Humanities Press, 1978), pp. 95–125.
150. IR (1895): xiii; Urquhart and Buckley, *Historical Statistics of Canada,* 16; IR (1898): xv.

151. Recent historiography has conclusively demonstrated, for widely separated locations and periods, the crucial role played by the family in initiating committal. See Richard Fox, *So Far Disordered in the Mind: Insanity in California, 1870–1930* (Berkeley, Calif.: University of California Press, 1978), p. 84; Finnane, *Insanity and the Insane*, 162–3; Nancy Tomes, "The Burden of Being Their Keepers: Patterns of Commitment to a Private Mental Hospital, 1840–1880," paper presented to the annual meeting of the Organization of American Historians, Detroit, 1981, pp. 7–11, 20; Scull, *Museums of Madness*, 240.

152. Occupational data is found in ARMS (1899): 53–4. For remaining sources, see Table 7. A similar sketch of the patient population at another Ontario asylum, Mimico, confirms these generalizations. See B. Willer and G. Miller, "Classification, Cause, and Symptoms of Mental Illness, 1890–1900 in Ontario," *Canadian Psychiatric Association Journal* 22, no. 5 (Aug. 1977): 232. That asylums were not geriatric institutions, as contemporaries alleged, is clear from such recent studies as Finnane, *Insanity and the Insane*, 130; Rosenkrantz and Vinovskis, "Invisible Lunatics," 99.

153. For example, Fox, *Disordered in the Mind*, 105, has used statistics to control for age so as to dispel the popular notion that the foreign-born were present in disproportionate numbers in American asylums. Cf. David Rothman, *The Discovery of the Asylum: Social Order and Disorder in the New Republic* (Boston, Mass.: Little, Brown, 1971), p. 283.

154. See Brown, "Living with God's Afflicted," 221, 266, 282–3; IC: vol. 17: Margaret V. to J. W. Langmuir, 10 Feb. 1882, describing some differences between Toronto and London Asylums for pay patients.

155. See above, note 77, and IR (1876): 22–3.

156. Ontario Archives: R.G.10, 20-C-4, London Asylum, Multipurpose Register, n.p., height and weight statistics for male admissions, Jan. 1–Dec. 3, 1901. Compare with contemporary normal values in C. M. Tidy, *Legal Medicine*, vol. 1 (New York: William Wood, 1882), pp. 145–7.

157. IC: vol. 16: R. A. Peacock to S. A. Armstrong, 16 Sept. 1907; IR: 1879; Urquhart and Buckley, *Historical Statistics of Canada*, 95.

158. IR (1866): 31–3.

159. IC: vol. 13: J. W. Langmuir to R. Mathison, 1 May 1877; ibid.: vol. 40: Robert C. to C. Sippi, 1 June 1891.

160. Ibid.: vol. 18: Thomas Short, Certificate re. Rebecca E., 8 March 1881; Robert Jones to J. W. Langmuir, 26 March 1881; Langmuir to Short, 18 March 1881.

161. Ibid.: vol. 67: Robert Christie to the Provincial Secretary, 5 March 1896. The negative response is written across the bottom of the letter.

162. Ibid.: vol. 16: John B. to R. M. Bucke, 21 Jan. 1880. The asylum agreed to care for the child. See ibid.: Bucke to J. W. Langmuir, 16 Jan. 1880 and Langmuir to Bucke, 28 Jan. 1880. Two other such cases arose in the next dozen years. See ibid.: vol. 67: Bucke to Robert Christie, 8 April 1892.

163. The same conclusion may have applied to at least some English asylums. See J. K. Walton, "Lunacy in the Industrial Revolution: A Study of Asylum Admissions in Lancashire, 1848–1850," *Journal of Social History* 13, no. 1 (1979): 12.

164. ARMS (1879): 330; IR (1882): 19.

165. ARMS (1870): 329.

166. *London (Ontario) Advertiser*, 8 Jan. 1879.

167. IR (1881): 32.

168. Ibid.: (1883): 53.

169. MSJ: 13 Feb. 1879. Bucke never made explicit the process or criteria by which patients were assigned to specific wards.

170. ARMS (1886): 26, (1877): 275–6. Some patients felt the diet inadequate. See IC: vol. 17: M. V. to J. W. Langmuir, 10 Feb. 1882.

171. See, for example, correspondence on patient Stephen F., in IC: vol. 18: R. M. Bucke, Discharge Certificate, 22 Aug. 1882; Stephen Lett to W. T. O'Reilly,

29 Aug. 1882; W. G. Metcalfe to O'Reilly, 29 Aug. 1882; O'Reilly to J. Russell, 30 April 1889.

172. IC: vol. 18: W. T. O'Reilly to Oliver Mowat, 12 March 1883.

173. See, for example, Erving Goffman, *Asylums: Essays on the Social Situation of Mental Patients and Other Inmates* (Garden City, N.Y.: Doubleday, 1961), pp. 218, 287–94.

174. IR (1879): 34, (1881): 31; IC: vol. 17: Bucke to J. W. Langmuir, 25 June 1881.

175. IR (1881): 33. In the first five years of Bucke's superintendency, he had two suicides and one homicide. See ARMS (1881): 357.

176. M.B. (25 April 1881): 130.

177. IC: vol. 17: J. B. to J. W. Langmuir, 2 Jan. 1881; ibid.: vol. 40: Petition re. James W. to Langmuir, n.d. (1878?); ibid.: vol. 18: W. S. W. to W. T. O'Reilly, 16 Oct. 1882.

178. IC: vol. 78: J. D. M. to Robert Christie, 19 June 1889; Bucke to Christie, 23 June 1899.

179. Ibid.: vol. 73: Bucke to Robert Christie, 22 Oct. 1898.

180. Ibid.: vol. 224: Robert Christie to Bucke, 8 Sept. 1897.

181. Ibid.: vol. 219: files for 1892 and 1897; ibid.: vol. 14: Bucke, Certificate, 7 Aug. 1877 re. escaped patient. Walt Whitman witnessed an attempted escape while on a visit with Bucke to the Hamilton Asylum: Walt Whitman, *Daybooks and Notebooks*, vol. 3, ed. William White (New York: New York University Press, 1978), 14 Aug. 1880.

182. See, for example, ARMS (1880): 327, (1890): 87.

183. IC: vol. 229: Bucke to J. W. Langmuir, 29 Nov. 1877; Langmuir to Bucke, 3 Dec. 1877; D. F. J. to Langmuir, 27 April 1880.

184. J. C. Bucknill and D. H. Tuke, *A Manual of Psychological Medicine* (Philadelphia, Penn.: Blanchard and Lea, 1858; reprinted New York: Hafner Publishing, 1968), p. 261. On the abuse of such statistics so as to suggest high cure rates, see Pliny Earle, *The Curability of Insanity: A Series of Studies* (Philadelphia, Penn.: J. B. Lippincott, 1887).

185. Sources as in Table 2.11.

186. ARMS (1880): 322, (1890): 82, (1900): 52. See also Ontario Archives: R.G.10, 20-C-3, vol. 12: "Register of Deaths, 1890–1915," which confirms the published reports.

187. While the social character of the asylum has been analyzed by few historians, other scholars have accorded it considerable attention. See, for example, William Caudill, *The Psychiatric Hospital as a Small Society* (Cambridge, Mass.: Harvard University Press, 1958); Goffman, *Asylums;* David Vail and Louis Miller, *Dehumanization and the Institutional Career* (Springfield, Ill.: Charles C. Thomas, 1966); Robert Perrucci, *Circle of Madness: On Being Insane and Institutionalized in America* (Englewood Cliffs, N.J.: Prentice-Hall, 1974).

CHAPTER 3   *Toward a secular physiology of mind*

1. Frank Turner, "The Victorian Conflict between Science and Religion: A Professional Dimension," *Isis* 69 (1978): 356–76; L. S. Jacyna, "Scientific Naturalism in Victorian Britain: An Essay in the Social History of Ideas" (Ph.D. dissertation, University of Edinburgh, 1980).

2. MUA, "McGill University Register of Matriculations no. 1, 1843–1893," 27 Nov. 1858. Two other matriculants listed their religion as Universalist. That McGill at this time was "an undenominational college of broadly Protestant character" is suggested in Stanley B. Frost, *McGill University for the Advancement of Learning*, vol. 1 (Montreal: McGill-Queen's University Press, 1980), p. 157. The Register of Matriculations records no religion beside the names of a small scattering of students.

3. Fred Landon, *Western Ontario and the American Frontier* (Toronto: McClelland

and Stewart, 1967 [1941]), pp. 115–16, 172–3; *Gospel Messenger or Universalist Advocate* 1 (January 1849): 8; Louis Foulds, *Universalists in Ontario* (Olinda, Ontario: Unitarian Universalist Church of Olinda, 1980) ch. 1 and ch. 2; Canada Census Returns, 1842: Canada West: London District, Township of London, microfilm reel C 1345; MUA, "McGill University Register of Matriculations," Edward Horatio Bucke, 12 Nov. 1850 and Augustus Henry Bucke, 21 Nov. 1851.

4. See Richard Eddy, *A History of Universalism* (New York: Christian Literature Company, 1894), pp. 440–2; David A. Johnson, *To Preach and Fight* (Tucson, Ariz.: Philomath Press, 1973); RMBC, 45 letters from Grosh to Bucke, 1857–1882.

5. Geoffrey Rowell, "The Origins and History of Universalist Societies in Britain, 1750–1850," *Journal of Ecclesiastical History* 22, no. 1 (1971): 35–6; George H. Williams, "American Universalism: A Bicentennial Historical Essay," *The Journal of the Universalist Historical Society* 9 (1971): especially 1–62. See also Stephen A. Marini, *Radical Sects of Revolutionary New England* (Cambridge, Mass.: Harvard University Press, 1982), ch. 4 and ch. 8.

6. Eddy, *History of Universalism*, 410, 412, 429; Ernest Cassara, ed., *Universalism in America, A Documentary History* (Boston, Mass.: Beacon Press, 1971), pp. 13, 16, 21; Rowell, "Universalist Societies in Britain," 38–42; Williams, "American Universalism," 11.

7. Williams, "American Universalism," 11–12; Cassara, *Universalism in America*, 6; Robert T. Handy, *A History of the Churches in the United States and Canada* (New York: Oxford University Press, 1977), p. 337. In fact, it would appear that in England the early Universalists were viewed as little better than infidels, (Rowell, "Universalist Societies in Britain," 43), while in America, though they claimed 800,000 adherents in 1851, opponents demanded that they be barred from jury service and schools (Cassara, *Universalism in America*, 29, 32).

8. Handy, *Churches in the United States and Canada*, 202, 337; Williams, "American Universalism," 12, 13, 50–2; Cassara, *Universalism in America*, 5, 20; Albert Post, *Popular Freethought in America, 1825–1850* (New York: Octagon Press, 1974 [1943]), pp. 226, 171, 195; Bucke wrote in *Cosmic Consciousness* (Secacus, N.J.: Citadel Press, 1977 [1901]), p. 3, that socialism was one of the three great revolutions of his age.

9. Ernest Cassara, "The Effect of Darwinism on Universalist Belief, 1860–1900," *Journal of the Universalist Historical Society* 1 (1959): 32–42; Williams, "American Universalism," 17.

10. R. Lawrence Moore, "Spiritualism," in *The Rise of Adventism: Religion and Society in Mid-Nineteenth-Century America*, ed. Edwin S. Gaustad (New York: Harper and Row, 1974), pp. 83, 87; Williams, "American Universalism," 2, 60; Rowell, "Universalist Societies in Britain," 36, 54.

11. Thomas Hall, *History of General Physiology* (Chicago: University of Chicago Press, 1969), vol. 1, ch. 18 and ch. 25; L. J. Rather, "G. E. Stahl's Psychological Physiology," *BHM* 35, no. 1 (1961): 37–49; Karl Figlio, "The Metaphor of Organization: An Historiographical Perspective on the Bio-Medical Sciences of the Early Nineteenth Century," *History of Science* 14 (1976): 25–7.

12. G. T. Goodfield, *The Growth of Scientific Physiology* (London: Hutchinson, 1960), pp. 13, 60–1; Everett Mendelsohn, "Physical Models and Physiological Concepts: Explanation in Nineteenth-Century Biology," *British Journal for the History of Science* 2, no. 7 (1965): 213.

13. June Goodfield-Toulmin, "Some Aspects of English Physiology: 1780–1840," *Journal of the History of Biology* 2, no. 2 (1969): 283–4; Hall, *History of General Physiology*, vol. 2: 220–2, 285–7.

14. Goodfield-Toulmin, "Aspects of English Physiology," 289, 286. On the debate in chemistry over the distinction between animate (organic) and inanimate (inorganic), see M. Teich, "On the Historical Foundations of Modern Bio-

chemistry," *Clio Medica* I (1965): 41–57. An essential context is provided in L. S. Jacyna, "Immanence or Transcendence: Theories of Life and Organization in Britain, 1790–1835," *Isis* 74 (Sept. 1983): 311–29.

15. Figlio, "Metaphor of Organization," 34–5; Goodfield-Toulmin, "Aspects of English Physiology," 290.

16. Figlio, "Metaphor of Organization," 272–7; Mendelsohn, "Physical Models and Physiological Concepts," 207, 212–13, 217–19; Goodfield, *Growth of Scientific Physiology*, 60, 75, 111; Oswei Temkin, "Basic Science, Medicine, and the Romantic Era," *BHM* 37, no. 2 (1963): 128.

17. Thomas Kuhn, "Energy Conservation as an Example of Simultaneous Discovery," in *Critical Problems in the History of Science*, ed. Marshall Claggett (Madison, Wis.: University of Wisconsin Press, 1959), p. 338; George Rosen, "The Conversion of Energy and the Study of Metabolism," in *The Historical Development of Physiological Thought*, eds. C. McC. Brooks and P. F. Cranefield (New York: Hafner, 1959), p. 245; P. M. Heimann, "Conversion of Forces and the Conservation of Energy," *Centaurus* 18 (1973–4): 147–61.

18. Vance Hall, "The Role of Force and Power in Liebig's Physiological Chemistry," *MH* 24, no. 1 (1980): 31, 38; W. R. Grove, *The Correlation of Physical Forces*, 3rd ed. (London: Longman, Brown, Green and Longmans, 1855 [1842]), pp. 15, 16, 190.

19. J. E. Carpenter, "Introductory Memoir," in W. B. Carpenter, *Nature and Man: Essays Scientific and Philosophical* (London: Kegan Paul, Trench, and Co., 1888), pp. 20–49.

20. W. B. Carpenter, "On the Mutual Relations of the Vital and Physical Forces," *Philosophical Transactions of the Royal Society of London* (1850): 752. On the later evolution of Carpenter's view of vital force, see Vance M. D. Hall, "The Contribution of the Physiologist William Benjamin Carpenter (1813–1885) to the Development of the Principles of the Correlation of Forces and the Conservation of Energy," *MH* 23, no. 2 (1979): 129–55.

21. R. M. Bucke, "Correlation of the Vital and the Physical Forces," *British American Journal* 3, 6, 7 and 8 (1862): 162–4; Carpenter, "Mutual Relations of the Vital and Physical Forces," 727–8.

22. Bucke, "Correlation of the Vital and the Physical Forces," 164–5; Carpenter, "Mutual Relations of the Vital and Physical Forces," 731; H. T. Buckle, *History of Civilization in England*, 1st American ed. from the 2nd London ed. (New York: D. Appleton, 1860), vol. 2, pp. 384–5.

23. Bucke, "Correlation of the Vital and the Physical Forces," 167, 193, 229, 166; Carpenter, "Mutual Relations of the Vital and Physical Forces," 733, 737, 738.

24. Bucke, "Correlation of the Vital and the Physical Forces," 225–9; Carpenter, "Mutual Relations of the Vital and Physical Forces," 740, 742, 744–6.

25. Bucke, "Correlation of the Vital and the Physical Forces," 195, 197; Carpenter, "Mutual Relations of the Vital and Physical Forces," 756.

26. Bucke, "Correlation of the Vital and the Physical Forces," 231–3; Carpenter, "Mutual Relations of the Vital and Physical Forces," 747–50.

27. Bucke, "Correlation of the Vital and the Physical Forces," 200. Carpenter, a devout Unitarian, appreciated the theological implications of his notion of correlated forces in a letter to Sir James Paget, reproduced in Carpenter, "Introductory Memoir," 53. Grove closed his published lectures by attributing a divine origin to indestructible force (Grove, *Correlation of Physical Forces*, 218). Similarly, Buckle was at pains to explain that science, by discovering the conservation of force, had actually revealed an even grander version of God's handiwork. (Buckle, *History of Civilization in England*, vol. 2: 385, 468–9.)

28. Harvey Cushing, *The Life of Sir William Osler* (London: Oxford University Press, 1940 [1925]), p. 85. This is not to suggest that interest in the correlation of forces suddenly disappeared. See E. L. Youmans, ed., *The Correlation and Conservation of Forces: A Series of Expositions* (New York: D. Appleton, 1865).

Bucke himself continued an interest in such topics and as late as 1870 was approached by an American publisher to consider revising his thesis for publication. See RMBC, Bucke to H. B. Forman, 9 Aug. 1870.

29. On these changes see Gerald Geison, *Michael Foster and the Cambridge School of Physiology* (Princeton, N.J.: Princeton University Press, 1978); R. D. French, "Some Problems and Sources in the Foundations of Modern Physiology in Great Britain," *History of Science* 10 (1971): 28–55; R. D. French, *Antivivisection and Medical Science in Victorian Society* (Princeton, N.J.: Princeton University Press, 1975) ch. 3; J. Schiller, "Physiology's Struggle for Independence in the First Half of the Nineteenth Century," *History of Science* 7 (1968): 64–89.

30. Carpenter uses this phrase to describe himself ("Mutual Relations of the Vital and Physical Forces," 753). It should be noted that for many years the most popular physiology text at McGill and elsewhere was W. G. Carpenter's *Principles of Human Physiology*, American ed. (Philadelphia, Penn.: Blanchard and Lea, 1855). It was used at McGill until at least 1872 (McCallum, "McGill Medical Faculty, 1847–1850," 171). The fragmentary evidence from extant annual calendars establishes that it was also used at Dalhousie University, from 1868 to 1884 (Dalhousie University Archives: Faculty of Medicine Calendars, 1868–1884), at Queen's University from 1861 to 1864 (Queen's University Archives: Faculty of Medicine Annual Announcement, 1861–1866), and at the Toronto School of Medicine from 1868 to 1887 (University of Toronto Archives: "Rules and Regulations for the Guidance of Students in Medicine," bound with the annual calendar, 1869–1887).

31. Goodfield, *Growth of Scientific Physiology*, 153–7.

32. RMBC, Diary (12 March 1863–7 Dec. 1864): 23 July, 23 Aug., 31 Aug. 1863. On Lewes as a Positivist popularizer, see W. M. Simon, *European Positivism in Nineteenth Century* (Ithaca, N.Y.: Cornell University Press, 1963), pp. 195–201.

33. Simon, *European Positivism*, 203; B. J. Paris, *Experiments in Life: George Eliot's Quest for Values* (Detroit, Mich.: Wayne State University Press, 1965).

34. RMBC, H. B. Forman to Bucke, 14 Oct. 1869, 1 July 1866, 28 June 1864, 29 April 1864, 16 March 1865, 21 Oct. 1866; Alfred Forman to Bucke, 1 Sept. 1864, 24 Oct. 1866, 24 Oct. 1873, 3 May 1875.

35. Diary (12 March 1863–7 Dec. 1864): 14 March 1863; Benjamin Ward Richardson, *Vita Medica: Chapters of Medical Life and Work* (London: Longmans, Green, 1897), p. 180; J. Russell Reynolds, "On the Relation of Practical Medicine to Philosophical Methods, and Popular Opinion," in his *Essays and Addresses* (London: Macmillan, 1896), pp. 5–7.

36. Diary (12 March 1863–7 Dec. 1864): 22 April, 23 April, 2 May, 27 May, 9 Sept., 10 Sept., 27 May, 3 Oct. 1863; RMBC, Diary (8 Dec. 1864–19 Oct. 1868): 6 March 1866.

37. Diary (12 March 1863–7 Dec. 1864): 3 May 1864; Diary (8 Dec. 1864–19 Oct. 1868): 21 Oct. 1865. Mill's article was entitled, "The Positivist Philosophy of Auguste Comte," *Westminister Review* 83 (April 1865): 161–92.

38. Diary (12 March 1863–7 Dec. 1864): 28 Nov. 1864; Diary (8 Dec. 1864–19 Oct. 1868): 21 Jan. 1867.

39. RMBC, Bucke to H. B. Forman, 1 April 1870; R. M. Bucke, *Man's Moral Nature: An Essay* (New York: G. P. Putnam's Sons, 1879), p. 2.

40. Bucke, *Cosmic Consciousness*, 7; Diary (12 March 1863–7 Dec. 1864): 23 July 1863; G. H. Lewes, *The Biographical History of Philosophy*, rev. ed. (New York: Appleton, 1859), pp. 778, *xxix*, 776, 779, 780, 783.

41. G. H. Lewes, *Comte's Philosophy of the Sciences* (London: Harry G. Bohn, 1853), p. *v*; Simon, *European Positivism*, 69–70. Another noted English physician-positivist is described in Susan Liveing, *A Nineteenth-Century Teacher, John Henry Bridges* (London: Kegan Paul, Trench, Trubner, 1926). Cf. Christopher Kent, *Brains and Numbers: Elitism, Comtism, and Democracy in Mid-Victorian England* (Toronto: University of Toronto Press, 1978) ch. 4, fn. 8.

42. Turner, "Victorian Conflict between Science and Religion."
43. Auguste Comte, *System of Positive Polity*, trans. J. H. Bridges (London: Green & Co., 1875 [1851]), vol. 1, p. 6.
44. Auguste Comte, *The Catechism of Positive Religion*, trans. Richard Congreve, 3rd ed. (London: Kegan Paul, Trench, Trubner, 1891 [1852]), pp. 41, 144–5, 155.
45. Ibid., 153, 176, 117; Auguste Comte, *System of Positive Polity*, trans. E. S. Beesley et al. (London: Longman's Green & Co., 1876 [1853]), vol. 3, pp. 528–9.
46. Diary (12 March 1863–7 Dec. 1864): 14 March 1863. Universalists eventually amalgamated with Unitarians, a denomination that revealed a marked receptivity to Positivism in contrast to other Protestant groups. See the two perceptive and complementary studies by Charles D. Cashdollar: "European Positivism and the American Unitarians," *Church History* 45, no. 4 (1976): 490–506, and "Auguste Comte and the American Reformed Theologians," *Journal of the History of Ideas* 39, no. 1 (1978): 61–79.
47. Auguste Comte, *System of Positive Polity*, trans. Frederic Harrison (London: Longmans, Green & Co., 1875 [1852]), vol. 2, p. 12; idem, *Catechism of Positive Religion*, 34, 45, 56, 41.
48. Lewes, *Biographical History of Philosophy*, 787; Simon, *European Positivism*, 48–9, 54–9; Cashdollar, "European Positivism and American Unitarians," passim.
49. RMBC, Bucke to H. B. Forman, 11 Dec. 1871.
50. Comte, *Catechism of Positive Religion*, 35, 176, 152, 177 (see also his Table C), 35, 36. On the general implications of Positivism's view of mind for psychology see Brian Mackenzie, "Darwinism and Positivism as Methodological Influences on the Development of Psychology," *Journal of the History of Behavioural Science* 12, no. 4 (1976): 330–7, and Kurt Danziger, "The Positivist Repudiation of Wundt," ibid., 153, no. 3 (1979): 205–30. Among others, J. S. Mill disagreed with Comte's refusal to make of psychology a separate science in his hierarchy. See Mill, "Positivist Philosophy of Auguste Comte," 174–7.
51. Comte, *Catechism of Positive Religion*, 6, 40, 119; idem, *System of Positive Polity*, vol. 1, p. 262.
52. J. C. Green, "Biology and Social Theory in the Nineteenth Century: Auguste Comte and Herbert Spencer," in Claggett, *Critical Problems in the History of Science*, 419–46; Barbara Haines, "The Inter-Relations between Social, Biological, and Medical Thought, 1750–1850: Saint-Simon and Comte," *British Journal for the History of Science* 11, no. 1 (1978): 19–35. Comte was not always consistent in his terminology, making the problem of assigning intellectual debts more complex. See Richard Vernon, "Auguste Comte and 'Development': A Note," *History and Theory* 17, no. 3 (1978): 323–6.
53. Cf. Rainer Baehre, "The Psychiatric Theory of Richard M. Bucke: A Study of the Impact of Evolutionary Naturalism on Psychiatric Thought in Late-Victorian Canada," paper presented to the Canadian Society for the History and Philosophy of Science, Saskatoon, Saskatchewan, June 1979. This paper is similar to the material found in Chapters 5 and 6 of his "From Pauper Lunatics to Bucke: Studies in the Management of Lunacy in Nineteenth-Century Ontario (M.Phil. thesis, University of Waterloo, 1976). As noted in Chapter 1, note 2, above, Bucke likely read Chamber's *Vestiges of the Natural History of Creation* (1844) at an early age. His diary (12 March 1863–7 Dec. 1864) first refers to the "developmental hypothesis" on 5 May 1863.
54. On Positivism in the United States see R. L. Hawkins, *Auguste Comte and the United States, 1816–1853* (Cambridge, Mass.: Harvard University Press, 1936) and idem, *Positivism in the United States, 1853–1861* (Cambridge, Mass.: Harvard University Press, 1938). In Canada, see J. A. Irving, "The Development of Philosophy in Central Canada from 1850 to 1900," *Canadian Historical Review* 31, no. 3 (1950): 252–87; A. B. McKillop, *A Disciplined Intelligence: Critical Inquiry and Canadian Thought in the Victorian Era* (Montreal: McGill-Queen's University Press, 1979), pp. 148–53; S. E. D. Shortt, *The Search for an Ideal:*

Six Canadian Intellectuals and their Convictions in an Age of Transition, 1890–1930
(Toronto: University of Toronto Press, 1976), Chapters 7 and 8.

55. Simon, *European Positivism*, 9.

56. RMBC, Bucke to H. B. Forman, 24 Nov. 1868, 19 Feb., 16 May 1869, 1 Feb.,
2 Oct. 1870.

57. Bucke, *Cosmic Consciousness*, 8.

58. Donal Sheehan, "Discovery of the Autonomic Nervous System," *Archives of
Neurology and Psychiatry* 35, no. 5 (1936): 1082–8; James C. White and Reginald
H. Smithwick, *The Autonomic Nervous System*, 2nd ed. (New York: Macmillan,
1941), pp. 7–8; Roger French, "The Origins of the Sympathetic Nervous System from Vesalius to Riolan," *MH* 15, no. 1 (1971): 45–54; Ruth Leys, "Background to the Reflex Controversy: William Alison and the Doctrine of Sympathy before Hall," in *Studies in the History of Biology*, eds. W. Coleman and C.
Limoges (Baltimore, Md.: Johns Hopkins University Press, 1980), vol. 4, pp.
1–66. On the social ramifications of the neurological concept of "sympathy",
see Christopher Lawrence, "The Nervous System and Society in the Scottish
Enlightenment," in *Natural Order: Historical Studies of Scientific Culture*, eds.
Barry Barnes and Steven Shapin (Beverly Hills, Calif.: Sage Publications,
1979), pp. 19–40. On the general history of the sympathetic system before 1800
see Richard Meier, " 'Sympathy' as a Concept in Early Neurophysiology,"
(Ph.D. dissertation, University of Chicago, 1979) and his, " 'Sympathy' in the
Neurophysiology of Thomas Willis," *Clio Medica* 17 (Dec. 1982): 95–111.

59. Erwin H. Ackerknecht, "The History of the Discovery of the Vegetative (Autonomic) Nervous System," *MH* 18, no. 1 (1974): 3, 4–5; Sheehan, "Discovery
of the Autonomic Nervous System," 1102–4; White and Smithwick, *Autonomic
Nervous System*, 11–13; W. Riese and E. C. Hoff, "A History of the Doctrine
of Cerebral Localization," *JHMAS* 6, no. 4 (1951): 467–70; G. H. Wang,
"Johann Paul Karplus (1866–1936) and Alois Kreidl (1864–1928): Two Pioneers
in the Study of Central Mechanisms of Vegetative Function," *BHM* 39, no. 6
(1965): 529–39.

60. Bucke, *Man's Moral Nature*, vii, ix; RMBC, Bucke to H. B. Forman, 11 Sept.
1871, 23 Dec. 1878.

61. RMBC, H. B. Forman to Bucke, 28 Nov. 1871. The works referred to are
J. G. Davey, *The Ganglionic Nervous System, Its Structure, Functions, and Diseases*
(London: John Churchill, 1858); Xavier Bichat, *Physiological Researches upon Life
and Death*, trans. Tobias Watkins, 1st American ed. from 2nd Paris ed. (Philadelphia, Penn.: Smith and Maxwell, 1809 [1800]). Richardson also mentioned
several minor articles and a chapter from Johannes Müller's *Handbook of Physiology* (1834–1840). A succinct summary of Richardson's views is found in his
Vita Medica, 381–3.

62. RMBC, Bucke to Forman, 18 June 1873, 27 June 1875. The book was Edward
Meryon, *On the Functions of the Sympathetic System of Nerves as a Physiological
Basis for a Rational System for Therapeutics* (London: J. & A. Churchill, 1872). It
was based on a series of articles appearing in the *Lancet* in 1871.

63. RMBC, Bucke to Forman, 15 March 1878. The work was likely A. Eulenburg
and P. Guttman, *Physiology and Pathology of the Sympathetic System of Nerves*,
trans. A. Napier (London: J. & A. Churchill, 1879). It had received the Astley
Cooper Prize for 1877 but the award was revoked when it was discovered that
dual authorship was apparently not permitted.

64. RMBC, Diary (1 Jan. 1878–19 Nov. 1878): 19 Feb., 4 Oct., 13 Nov. 1878.

65. RMBC, Bucke to H. B. Forman, 11 Dec. 1871.

66. RMBC, Bucke to H. B. Forman, 10 Dec. 1872, 17 Feb., 6 Oct. 1875; copies of
the address are referred to in H. B. Forman to Bucke, 20 Jan. 1876, and Biggs
Andrews to Bucke, 24 Dec. 1875.

67. R. M. Bucke, "The Functions of the Great Sympathetic Nervous System," *AJI*
34 (Oct. 1877): 115–59; idem, "The Moral Nature and the Great Sympathetic,"
AJI 35 (Oct. 1878): 229–53; RMBC, Bucke to H. B. Forman, 6 Nov. 1877, 27

Oct. 1878, and H. B. Forman to Bucke, 1 Jan. 1878. His decision to publish in book form is first announced to Forman in a letter of 29 July 1877.

68. RMBC, Bucke to H. B. Forman, 14 July 1878.

69. RMBC, Bucke to H. B. Forman, 27 Oct. 1877. See Benjamin Ward Richardson, *Diseases of Modern Life*, American edition (New York: D. Appleton, 1895 [1875]).

70. RMBC, Bucke to H. B. Forman, 17 April 1879, and Diary (1 Jan. 1878–19 Nov. 1878): 18 Nov. 1879.

71. Bucke, *Cosmic Consciousness*, 8; RMBC, Bucke to H. B. Forman, 11 April 1879.

72. RMBC, Bucke to H. B. Forman, 23 Dec. 1878; 26 Feb., (?) March, and 13 May 1879.

73. RMBC, H. B. Forman to Bucke, 22 April 1879, 24 June 1879.

74. RMBC, Bucke to H. B. Forman, 13 May 1879, 8 July 1879, 6 Jan. 1888; Statements of Account from G. P. Putnam, 1879, 1880, 1883; from Trubner and Company, 31 Dec. 1880; from Willing and Williamson, the Canadian agent, 1 Oct. 1880, 15 Nov. 1883; 119 copies were sold in the United States and 123 copies in Canada.

75. R. M. Young, *Mind, Brain, and Adaptation in the Nineteenth Century, Cerebral Localization and its Biological Context from Gall to Ferrier* (Oxford: Clarendon Press, 1970), pp. 210–20; W. Riese, *A History of Neurology* (New York: M. D. Publications, 1959) ch. 4; idem and E. C. Hoff, "A History of the Doctrine of Cerebral Localization," *JHMAS* 5, no. 1 (1959): 50–63.

76. Young, *Cerebral Localization and its Biological Context*, ch. 1; Erwin Ackerknecht, "Contributions of Gall and the Phrenologists to Knowledge of Brain Function," in *The History and Philosophy of Knowledge of the Brain and its Functions*, ed. F. N. L. Poynter (Oxford: Blackwell Scientific Publications, 1958), pp. 149–53.

77. Barbara Tizard, "Theories of Brain Localization from Flourens to Lashley," *MH* 3, no. 2 (1959): 132–9; A. E. Walker, "The Development of the Concept of Cerebral Localization in the Nineteenth Century," *BHM* 31, no. 2 (1957): 102–12; F. M. R. Walshe, "Some Reflections upon the Opening Phase of the Physiology of the Cerebral Cortex, 1850–1900," in Poynter, *Brain and its Functions*, 223–9; Francis Schiller, *Paul Broca, Founder of French Anthropology, Explorer of the Brain* (Berkeley, Calif.: University of California Press, 1979), ch. 10. On the unitary nature of higher functions and the "sensorium commune" in eighteenth century thought, see Karl Figlio, "Theories of Perception and the Physiology of Mind in the late Eighteenth Century," *History of Science* 12 (1975): 177–212.

78. Young, *Cerebral Localization and its Biological Context*, 214; Walshe, "Physiology of the Cerebral Cortex," 226–7; Tizard, "Theories of Brain Localization," 138–9.

79. Tizard, "Theories of Brain Localization," 138; Riese and Hoff, "Doctrine of Cerebral Localization," 64; H. T. Englehardt, "John Hughlings Jackson and the Mind–Body Relation," *BHM* 49, no. 2 (1975): 141–3.

80. Roger Smith, "The Background of Physiological Psychology in Natural Philosophy," *History of Science* 9 (1973): 87; Robert Hoeldtke, "The History of Associationism and British Medical Psychology," *MH* 11, no. 1 (1967): 46, 48.

81. See note 79 above and Smith, "Background of Physiological Psychology," 82–4.

82. RMBC, Diary (12 March 1863–7 Dec. 1864): 19 March 1863, 3 May, 5 July, 7 Nov., 28 Nov. 1864.

83. Ibid., 26 March 1863; RMBC, Bucke to H. B. Forman, 30 Nov. 1873.

84. Young, *Cerebral Localization and its Biological Context*, ch. 3 and 5; idem, "The Functions of the Brain from Gall to Ferrier (1808–1886)," *Isis* 59 (1968): 251–68; Smith, "Background of Physiological Psychology," 95–7, 100–1; Englehardt, "John Hughlings Jackson," 140–5.

85. Auguste Comte, *System of Positive Polity*, trans. Frederic Harrison (London: Longmans, Green & Co., 1875 [1852]), vol. 2, p. 357; Herbert Spencer, *Social Statics* (New York: Appleton, 1875 [1852]), pp. 31, 41–3; cf. Alexander Bain, *The Emotions and the Will*, 3rd ed. (London: Longmans, Green & Co., 1880 [1859]), p. 268.
86. Bucke, *Man's Moral Nature*, xi.
87. Geison, *Michael Foster*, ch. 2; French, *Foundations of Modern Physiology in Great Britain*, ch. 3; Lloyd G. Stevenson, "Anatomical Reasoning in Physiological Thought," in Brooks and Cranefield, *Historical Development of Physiological Thought*, 27–38.
88. Bucke, *Man's Moral Nature*, 52; Meryon, *Functions of the Sympathetic System*, 11.
89. Bucke, *Man's Moral Nature*, 113.
90. Bucke, *Man's Moral Nature*, 128–49, discussed Bacon, judging him "perhaps the greatest intellect the world has seen" (149). He was convinced that Bacon was the true author of Shakespeare's work. He became obsessed with this idea, writing to Harry Forman (RMBC, 8 Jan. 1900) of his discovery, "I am afraid of my life that some other man will get on to the track and cut me out! And I very much want to have the credit of the discovery for myself." On this topic he published two essays in the *Canadian Magazine* – 9 (Sept. 1897): 363–78, 14 (January 1900): 272–5 – as well as brief pieces in the *Conservator* 10 (November 1899): 138, 12 (July 1901): 74–5.
91. Davey, *Ganglionic Nervous System*, 80; Carpenter, *Principles of Human Physiology*, 575, 580; Comte, *System of Positive Polity*, vol. 1: 575; Alexander Bain, *The Senses and the Intellect*, 3rd ed. (London: Longmans, Green & Co., 1868 [1855]), ch. 3 and ch. 4.
92. Bucke, *Man's Moral Nature*, 13, 16, 19, 20, 22, 33, 34.
93. RMBC, Diary (12 March 1863–19 Oct. 1864): 19 March 1863; Alexander Bain, "Critical Notice" of *Man's Moral Nature* in *Mind* 5 (Oct. 1880): 559–62.
94. Bucke, *Man's Moral Nature*, 25.
95. Ibid., 55, 57, 58, 64. That others write in a similar fashion is clear from Davey, *Ganglionic Nervous System*, 114, 219, 265; Meryon, *Functions of the Sympathetic System*, 21, 26, 27, 40; W. B. Carpenter, *Principles of Mental Physiology* (New York: Appleton, 1874), p. 129.
96. Bucke, *Man's Moral Nature*, x.
97. Ibid., 47.
98. Comte, *Catechism of Positive Religion*, 177, Table C idem, *System of Positive Polity*, trans. Richard Congreve (London: Longmans, Green, 1877 [1854]), vol. 4, pp. 209–12; cf. Comte, *System of Positive Polity*, vol. 1, p. 551. See above, note 61.
99. Bichat, *Physiological Researches*, 54, 56, 61. On Bichat see W. R. Albury, "Experiment and Explanation in the Physiology of Bichat and Magendie," in *Studies in the History of Biology*, eds. W. Coleman and C. Limoges (Baltimore, Md.: Johns Hopkins University Press, 1977), vol. 1, pp. 47–131; C. Haywood, "D. H. Lawrence's 'Blood-Consciousness' and the Work of Xavier Bichat and Marshall Hall," *Etudes Anglaises* 32, no. 4 (1979): 397–413.
100. Davey, *Ganglionic Nervous System*, 80–1; Daniel Hack Tuke, *Illustrations of the Influence of the Mind upon the Body in Health and Disease*, 2nd ed. (London: J. & A. Churchill, 1884 [1872]), vol. 1, p. 166; Bain, " 'Critical Notice' of *Man's Moral Nature*," 561. If Bichat's views on the sympathetic nerves were anachronistic by the 1870s, they had enjoyed currency in popular American physiology during the 1830s. See Stephen Nissenbaum, *Sex, Diet, and Debility in Jacksonian America: Sylvester Graham and Health Reform* (Westport, Conn.: Greenwood Press, 1980), pp. 62–4.
101. Bain, " 'Critical Notice' of *Man's Moral Nature*," 561; Bucke, *Man's Moral Nature*, 65, 87. See Elizabeth Fee, "Nineteenth-Century Craniology: The Study of the Female Skull," *BHM* 53, no. 3 (1979): 415–33. On women as repositories of morality, see Barbara Welter, "The Cult of True Womanhood: 1820–

1860," *American Quarterly* 18, no. 2 (1966): 151–74; Carroll Smith-Rosenberg and Charles Rosenberg, "The Female Animal: Medical and Biological Views of Woman and Her Role in Nineteenth-Century America," *Journal of American History* 60, no. 2 (1973): 332–56.

102. Bucke, *Man's Moral Nature*, 65, 67–70, 74, 76, 96, 101. Carpenter drew an analogous correspondence between intellect and brain volume, *Human Physiology*, 533.

103. Bucke, *Man's Moral Nature*, 134–5. This view he would have found in many sources but certainly in Carpenter, *Human Physiology*, 835.

104. Bucke, *Man's Moral Nature*, 134; Comte, *Catechism of Positive Religion*, 199. Bucke made extensive use of Haeckel's approach in "The Origins of Insanity," *AJI* 49 (July 1892): 56–66. For a survey of recapitulation see Robert E. Grinder, *A History of Genetic Psychology: The First Science of Human Development* (New York: John Wiley and Sons, 1967), Part III, "The Theory of Recapitulation," pp. 89–132.

105. Bain, *Emotions and the Will*, 55; Comte, *Catechism of Positive Religion*, 158; Carpenter, *Principles of Mental Physiology*, 107–8.

106. Bucke, *Man's Moral Nature*, 37, 38, 159–61.

107. Ibid., 162, 184.

108. Comte, *System of Positive Polity*, vol. 1: 229, 234; Bucke, *Man's Moral Nature*, 169–74.

109. Bucke, *Man's Moral Nature*, 191, 198–200; Comte, *System of Positive Polity*, 17, 24; Carpenter, *Principles of Mental Physiology*, 107; Bain, *Emotions and the Will*, 271.

110. RMBC, Bucke to H. B. Forman, 27 Nov. 1878, 27 May, 19 Aug. 1879; Alfred Forman to Bucke, 24 Oct. 1879; H. B. Forman to Bucke, 17 Oct. 1879; Edward Carpenter to Bucke, 28 May 1881.

111. Horace Traubel, *With Walt Whitman in Camden* (New York: Rowman and Littlefield, 1961 [1907]), vol. 2, p. 179: 22 Aug. 1888.

112. *Alienist and Neurologist* 1 (July 1880): 393; *AJI* 36 (April 1880): 532.

113. *AJI* 36 (April 1880): 533; *Mind* 5 (January 1880): 151. Not all reviewers were hostile. See W. D. Le Sueur in *Rose-Belford's Canadian Monthly and National Review*, n.s., 3 (July 1879): 104–5. The latter shared with Bucke an interest in both Positivism and evolution. See McKillop, *Disciplined Intelligence*, ch. 5.

114. Kent, *Brains and Numbers*, 56–7; Michael McCormick, "The Biological Theory of Auguste Comte," (Ph.D. dissertation, University of Texas at Austin, 1976), pp. 5–8.

115. Charles Rosenberg, *No Other Gods: On Science and American Social Thought* (Baltimore, Md.: Johns Hopkins University Press, 1976), p. 3.

116. R. M. Young, "Natural Theology, Victorian Periodical, and the Fragmentation of the Common Context," in *Darwin to Einstein: Historical Studies on Science and Belief,* eds. Colin Chant and John Fauvel (Burnt Mill, Harlow: Longman in association with the Open University Press, 1976), pp. 69–107.

117. Sally Kohlstedt, *The Formation of the American Scientific Community: The American Association for the Advancement of Science, 1848–1860* (Urbana, Ill.: University of Illinois Press, 1976), pp. 132–3; G. H. Daniels, "The Process of Professionalization in American Science: The Emergent Period, 1820–1860," *Isis* 58 (1967): 157–66; Susan F. Cannon, *Science in Culture: The Early Victorian Period* (New York: Dawson and Science History Publications, 1978); Roy MacLeod, "Resources of Science in Victorian England: The Endowment of Science Movement, 1868–1900," in *Science and Society, 1600–1900*, ed. Peter Mathias (New York: Cambridge University Press, 1972), pp. 111–66.

118. Frank Turner, "Rainfall, Plagues, and the Prince of Wales: A Chapter in the Conflict of Religion and Science," *Journal of British Studies* 13 (May 1974): 46–65; idem, "Victorian Conflict between Science and Religion."

119. Geison, *Michael Foster;* E. C. Atwater, " 'Squeezing Mother Nature': Experimental Physiology in the United States Before 1870," *BHM* 52, no. 2 (1978):

326–7; L. S. Jacyna, "The Physiology of Mind, the Unity of Nature, and the Moral Order in Victorian Thought," *British Journal for the History of Science* 14, no. 47 (1981): 109–32.

120. This theme was the focus of George Rosen's prescient "Political Order and Human Health in Jeffersonian Thought," *BHM* 26, no. 1 (1952): 32–44, and has more recently been explored in Roger Cooter's perceptive "The Power of the Body: The Early Nineteenth Century," in Barnes and Shapin, *Natural Order*, 73–92.

121. This process was particularly evident in American public health organizations where, by 1880, laypeople had been almost entirely displaced by physicians. See Barbara Rosenkrantz, "Cart before Horse: Theory, Practice and Professional Image in American Public Health, 1870–1920," *JHMAS* 29, no. 1 (1974): 57–9, 61, and John Duffy, "The American Medical Profession and Public Health: From Support to Ambivalence," *BHM* 53, no. 1 (1979): 1, 7–8.

122. Burton Bledstein, *The Culture of Professionalism: The Middle Class and the Development of Higher Education in America* (New York: W. W. Norton, 1976), p. 90.

123. M. Jeanne Peterson, *The Medical Profession in Mid-Victorian London* (Berkeley, Calif.: University of California Press, 1978), p. 286.

CHAPTER 4 *The social genesis of etiological speculation*

1. W. F. Bynum, "Rationales for Therapy in British Psychiatry: 1780–1834," *MH* 18, no. 4 (1974): 324; Andrew Scull, *Museums of Madness: The Social Organization of Insanity in Nineteenth-Century England* (London: Allen Lane, 1979), pp. 125–40; idem, "The Domestication of Madness," *MH* 27, no. 3 (1983): 233–48; Roger Cooter, "Phrenology and British Alienists, c. 1825–1845, Part I: Converts to a Doctrine," *MH* 20, no. 1 (1976): 3.

2. W. B. Carpenter, *Principles of Mental Physiology* (New York: Appleton, 1874), p. 2; J. C. Bucknill and D. H. Tuke, *A Manual of Psychological Medicine* (Philadelphia, Penn.: Blanchard and Lea, 1858 [reprinted New York: Hafner, 1968]), p. 345; Henry Maudsley, *Pathology of Mind* (London: Macmillan, 1879), p. 86. All italics in the original works.

3. Bucknill and Tuke, *Manual of Psychological Medicine*, 51, 187. See David Rothman, *The Discovery of the Asylum: Social Order and Disorder in the New Republic* (Boston, Mass.: Little, Brown, 1971), ch. 5; Charles Rosenberg, *The Trial of the Assassin Guiteau: Psychiatry and Law in the Gilded Age* (Chicago: University of Chicago Press, 1968), pp. 67–70. Norman Dain, *Concepts of Insanity in the United States, 1789–1865* (New Brunswick, N.J.: Rutgers University Press 1964), pp. 85–108.

4. S. P. Fullwinder, "Insanity as Loss of Self: The Moral Insanity Controversy Revisited," *BHM* 41, no. 1 (1975): 97.

5. Bucknill and Tuke, *Manual of Psychological Medicine*, 351, 353–5, 366–7, 376–7. See also D. H. Tuke, *Illustrations of the Influence of the Mind upon the Body in Health and Disease*, 2nd ed. (London: J. & A. Churchill, 1884 [1872]), vol. 1, p. 122.

6. Bucknill and Tuke, *Manual of Psychological Medicine*, 367, 343. Carpenter held similar views on cerebral nutrition. See W. B. Carpenter, *Principles of Human Physiology* (Philadelphia, Penn.: Blanchard and Lea, 1855), p. 628.

7. Nathan G. Hale inexplicably identifies somatic psychiatry with post-1865 neurologists and apparently fails to appreciate it as much older tradition. See his *Freud and the Americans: The Beginnings of Psychoanalysis in the United States 1896–1917* (New York: Oxford University Press, 1971), ch. 3 and ch. 4.

8. Ruth B. Caplan, *Psychiatry and the Community in Nineteenth-Century America* (New York: Basic Books, 1969), pp. 126, 131; Norman Dain, *Concepts of Insanity*, 108–113. Caplan (131) and other scholars, such as Norman Dain and Eric Carlson in "Moral Insanity in the United States, 1835–1866," *American Journal of Psychiatry* 118 (March 1962): 799, incorrectly imply an inherent an-

tagonism between somatic pathology and psychological etiology. A concise corrective is found in L. S. Jacyna, "Somatic Theories of Mind and the Interests of Medicine in Britain, 1850–1879," *MH* 26, no. 3 (1982): 233.

9. John Conolly, *An Inquiry Concerning the Indications of Insanity* (London: John Taylor, 1830 [reprinted London: Dawsons, 1964]), ch. 4 and ch. 5; George Man Burrows, *Commentaries on the Causes, Forms Symptoms, and Treatment, Moral and Medical, of Insanity* (London: Thomas and George Underwood, 1828), ch. 4. On the appearance of the idea of hereditary degeneration in very early nineteenth-century views of insanity see Michael Donnelly, *Managing the Mind, A Study of Medical Psychology in Early Nineteenth-Century Britain* (London: Tavistock Publications, 1983), pp. 121, 134.

10. Maudsley, *Pathology of Mind*, 84.

11. Henry Maudsley, "Insanity," in *A System of Medicine*, ed. J. Russell Reynolds (Philadelphia, Penn.: Henry C. Lea's Sons, 1880), vol. 1, p. 55; Isaac Ray, *Mental Hygiene* (Boston, Mass.: Ticknor and Fields 1863 [reprinted New York: Hafner, 1968]), p. 18.

12. Charles Rosenberg, "The Place of George M. Beard in Nineteenth-Century Psychiatry," *BHM* 36, no. 3 (1962): 245–9. See also Barbara Sicherman, "The Uses of a Diagnosis: Doctors, Patients, and Neurasthenia," *JHMAS* 32, no. 1 (1977): 33–54.

13. The trend toward biological reductionism in the 1880s is discussed in Charles Rosenberg, "The Bitter Fruit: Heredity, Disease, and Social Thought in Nineteenth-Century America," *Perspectives in American History* (Cambridge, Mass.: Harvard University Press, 1974), vol. 8, pp. 189–235. This hereditarianism, not somaticism, was what congealed in the psychiatric thought of the 1870s. Cf. Hale, *Freud and the Americans*, ch. 3. On British somaticism in the 1870s, see Michael Clark, "The Rejection of Psychological Approaches to Mental Disorder in Late Nineteenth-Century British Psychiatry," in *Madhouses, Mad-Doctors, and Madmen: The Social History of Psychiatry in the Victorian Era*, ed. Andrew Scull (Philadelphia, Penn.: University of Pennsylvania Press, 1981), pp. 271–312.

14. E. C. Spitzka, *Insanity: Its Classification, Diagnosis, and Treatment* (New York: E. B. Treat, 1889), p. 369.

15. For example, see the popular text by Henry J. Berkley, *A Treatise on Mental Disease* (New York: D. Appleton, 1900), pp. 52–3.

16. R. M. Bucke, "Mental Evolution in Man," *British Medical Journal* 2 (11 Sept. 1897): 643. (Printed also in the *Journal of the American Medical Association* 29 (23 Oct. 1897): 821–4.) This paper, Bucke's Presidential Address to the Psychological Section, British Medical Association, provoked critical editorial commentary in the *British Medical Journal* [2 (25 Sept. 1897): 827–8] and several hostile letters [2 (9 Oct. 1897): 1030, and 2 (3 Oct. 1897): 1298–9].

17. R. M. Bucke, "The Origins of Insanity," *AJI* 49 (July 1892): 61.

18. R. M. Bucke, "Cosmic Consciousness," *Proceedings of the American Medico-Psychological Association* 1 (1894): 327. See, for example, Charles Darwin, *The Expression of Emotions in Man and Animals* (London: John Murray, 1872) and G. J. Romanes, *Mental Evolution in Animals* (New York: Appleton, 1884).

19. R. M. Bucke, "The Growth of the Intellect," *AJI* 39 (July 1882): 40–1, in which he cites Charles Lyell's *The Geological Evidences for the Antiquity of Man* (London: John Murray, 1863).

20. Ibid., 39. See Max Müller, *Lectures on the Science of Languages*, 2nd rev. ed. (New York: Charles Scribner, 1866), vol. 1, pp. 353–4, 356; idem, *The Science of Thought* (New York: Charles Scribner's Sons, 1887), vol. 1, pp. 81–2. On Müller and his contemporary colleagues, see S. J. Schmidt, "German Philosophy of Language in the Late Nineteenth-Century," in *History of Linguistic Thought and Contemporary Linguistics*, ed. Herman Parret (Berlin: Walter de Gruyter, 1976), pp. 658–84.

21. Bucke, "Growth of the Intellect," 41.

22. Noted in Hans Aarsleff, *The Study of Language in England, 1780–1860* (Princeton, N.J.: Princeton University Press, 1967), p. 223.

23. George John Romanes, *Mental Evolution in Man: Origin of Human Faculty* (London: Kegan Paul and Trench, 1888), especially pp. 238, 343, 354–7. On Romanes, see the essay by John E. Leach in *Dictionary of Scientific Biography*, ed. C. C. Gillispie (New York: Charles Scribner's Sons, 1975), vol. 11, pp. 516–20; F. M. Turner, *Between Science and Religion: The Reaction to Scientific Naturalism in Late Victorian England* (New Haven, Conn.: Yale University Press, 1974), ch. 6.

24. Müller, *Science of Languages*, vol. 1: 31, 24.

25. Bucke, "Origins of Insanity," 59.

26. Auguste Comte, *The Catechism of Positive Religion*, trans. Richard Congreve, 3rd ed. (London: Kegan Paul, Trench, Trubner, 1891 [1852]), p. 199; idem, *System of Positive Polity*, trans. by John Henry Bridges (London: Longmans, Green & Co., 1875 [1851]), vol. 1, p. 263; Herbert Spencer, *The Principles of Biology*, rev. ed. (New York: Appleton, 1898 [1864]), vol. 1, p. 453.

27. The derivation and nineteenth-century flowering of recapitulation theory are described perceptively by Stephen Jay Gould, *Ontogeny and Phylogeny* (Cambridge, Mass.: Harvard University Press, 1977), Part I. Note also William Coleman, "Limits of Recapitulation Theory: Carl Friedrich Kielmeyer's Critique of the Presumed Parallelism of Earth History, Ontogeny, and the Present Order of Organism," *Isis* 64 (Sept. 1973): 341–50, and R. G. Rinard, "The Problem of the Organic Individual: Ernst Haeckel and the Development of the Biogenetic Law," *Journal of the History of Biology* 14, no. 2 (1981): 249–75.

28. Bucke, "Origins of Insanity," 58.

29. On Haeckel, see Gould, *Ontogeny and Phylogeny*, 76–114; Jane Oppenheimer, "Recapitulation," in *Dictionary of the History of Ideas*, ed. P. P. Weiner (New York: Charles Scribner's Sons, 1973), vol. 4, pp. 56–9; George Uschmann, essay on Haeckel in Gillispie, *Dictionary of Scientific Biography*, vol. 6: 6–11.

30. Bucke, "Origins of Insanity," 59. An earlier statement of recognition appears in Bucke, "Growth of the Intellect," 46. Maudsley, *Pathology of Mind*, 102.

31. Bucke, "Origins of Insanity," 61.

32. Bucke, "Growth of the Intellect," 48–52. See Lazarus Geiger, *Contribution to the History of the Development of the Human Race: Lectures and Dissertations*, trans. David Asher (London: Trubner, 1880), esp. pp. 49–62. Geiger accepted recapitulation theory.

33. Bucke, "Origins of Insanity," 64, 62–3.

34. Ibid., 65.

35. Bucke, "Mental Evolution in Man," 645.

36. R. M. Bucke, "The Function of the Great Sympathetic Nervous System," *AJI* 34 (Oct. 1877): 132.

37. R. M. Bucke, "Value of the Study of Medicine," *Montreal Medical Journal* 20 (Nov. 1891): 339–40; idem, "Origins of Insanity," 60.

38. R. M. Bucke, testimony, *Report of the Commission Appointed to Enquire into the Prison and Reformatory System of the Province of Ontario, Ontario Sessional Papers* (1891), pp. 531, 534. See also ARMS (1882): 353–4.

39. *Report of Prison and Reformatory System of Ontario*, 531. Bucke believed that some of the insane were "conceived under certain conditions" which led to later imperfections. This was a "congenital" as opposed to "hereditary" cause. The intoxication of a parent would serve as as example.

40. Ibid., 532.

41. Gould, *Ontogeny and Phylogeny*, 115; Robert E. Grinder, *A History of Genetic Psychology* (New York: W. W. Norton, 1967), p. 91.

42. Gould, *Ontogeny and Phylogeny*, 77.

43. Ibid., 117, 132.

44. Sigmund Freud, *Introductory Lectures on Psychoanalysis* (London: George Allen and Unwin, 1961), p. 199.

45. Gould, *Ontogeny and Phylogeny*, 156–7; Frank Sulloway, *Freud: Biologist of the Mind* (New York: Basic Books, 1979), pp. 199–204, 258–61, 398–9.
46. Dorothy Ross, G. *Stanley Hall: The Psychologist as Prophet* (Chicago: University of Chicago Press, 1972), esp. ch. 6; Charles Strickland, "The Child and the Race: The Doctrine of Recapitulation and Culture Epochs in the Rise of the Child-Centered Ideal in American Educational Thought," (Ph.D. dissertation, University of Wisconsin, 1963), ch. 4 and ch. 7; S. L. Schlossman, "G. Stanley Hall and the Boys' Club: Conservative Applications of Recapitulation Theory," *Journal of the History of Behavior Science* 9 (April 1973): 140–7; Gould, *Ontogeny and Phylogeny*, 147–55.
47. Grinder, *History of Genetic Psychology*, 92; Oppenheimer, "Recapitulation,"; Gould, *Ontogeny and Phylogeny*, 131.
48. Marvin Wolfgang, "Cesare Lombroso, 1835–1901," in *Pioneers in Criminology*, ed. Hermann Mannheim (Montclair, N.J.: Paterson Smith, 1972), p. 244; Gould, *Ontogeny and Phylogeny*, 120–5; idem, *The Mismeasure of Man* (New York: W. W. Norton, 1981), pp. 122–42.
49. Jacques Moreau de Tours, *Un Chapître Oublié de la Pathologie Mentale* (Paris: Masson, 1850), p. 18.
50. Prosper Lucas, *Traité Philosophique et Physiologique de l'Hérédité Naturelle dans les Estates de Santé et de Maladie du Systèm Nerveux* (Paris: J.-B. Bailliere, 1847–50), vol. 2, p. 534.
51. B. A. Morel, *Traité des Dégénérescences Physiques, Intéllectuals, et Morales de l'Espèce Humaine et des Causes qui Produisent ces Variétés Maladies* (Paris: J.-B. Bailliere, 1857), pp. 6, 70. His *Traité des Maladies Mentales* (Paris: Masson, 1860) first introduced the law of progressivity. See also Ruth Friedländer, "Benedict-Augustin Morel and the Development of the Theory of Degenerescence," (Ph.D. dissertation, University of California, 1973) and Jan Goldstein, "French Psychiatry in Social and Political Context: The Formation of the New Profession, 1820–1860," (Ph.D. dissertation, Columbia University, 1978), esp. ch. 5.
52. V. Magnan and P. Legrain, *Les Dégénérés (Etat Mental et Syndromes Episodiques)* (Paris: Rueff, 1895), p. 44.
53. No adequate English-language sources discuss medical degeneration theory, but see E. H. Ackerknect, *A Short History of Psychiatry*, trans. Sula Wolff (New York: Hafner, 1968), ch. 7; Milton Gold, "The Early Psychiatrists on Degeneration and Genius," *Psychoanalysis and Psychoanalytic Review* 47, no. 4 (1960): 37–55; Hale, *Freud and the Americans*, 76–83; Colin Martindale, "Degeneration, Disinhibition, and Genius," *Journal of the History of Behavior Science* 7, no. 2 (1971): 177–82; Rosenberg, "Bitter Fruit," 217–25; Richard Walter, "What Became of the Degenerate? A Brief History of a Concept," *JHMAS* 11, no. 4 (1956): 422–9; Henry Werlinder, *Psychopathy: A History of the Concepts* (Uppsala: Uppsala University, 1978), ch. 4; Robert A. Nye, *Crime, Madness, and Politics in Modern France, The Medical Concept of National Decline* (Princeton, N.J.: Princeton University Press, 1984), ch. 4 and ch. 5.
54. Max Nordeau, *Degeneration*, reprint ed. (New York: Howard Fertig, 1968 [1895]); Richard Dugdale, *The Jukes: A Study in Crime, Pauperism, Disease, and Heredity* (New York: G. P. Putnam's Press, 1877).
55. Christopher Hibbert, *The Roots of Evil* (London: Weidenfeld and Nicholson, 1963), p. 197; Joseph M. Hawes, *Children in Urban Society: Juvenile Delinquency in Nineteenth-Century America* (New York: Oxford University Press, 1971), pp. 248–58; M. S. W. Vince, "Gabriel Tarde, 1843–1904," in Mannheim, *Pioneers in Criminology*, 292–304.
56. On Lombroso see note 48 above, and the following: Hawes, *Children in Urban Society*, ch. 11; Hibbert, *Roots of Evil*, part III; George Mora, "One Hundred Years from Lombroso's First Essay, Genius and Insanity," *American Journal of Psychiatry* 121 (Dec. 1964): 562–71.
57. Havelock Ellis, *The Criminal* (New York: Scribner and Welford, 1890); Robert

Fletcher, "The New School of Criminal Anthropology," *American Anthropologist* 4 (July 1891): 201–36; H. D. Way, "Criminal Anthropology," *Proceedings of the National Prison Association* (1890): 274–91.

58. August Drahms, *The Criminal* (New York: Macmillan, 1900); Arthur Mac-Donald, *Criminology* (New York: Funk and Wagnalls, 1893). An extensive discussion on Lombroso's influence in the United States is found in Arthur Fink, *Causes of Crime: Biological Theories in the United States 1800–1915* (New York: A. S. Barnes, 1962 [1938]).

59. See, for example, Mark Haller, *Eugenics: Hereditarian Attitudes in American Thought* (New Brunswick, N.J.: Rutgers University Press, 1963), ch. 2 and ch. 3; Donald Pickens, *Eugenics and the Progressives* (Nashville, Tenn.: Vanderbilt University Press, 1968), ch. 1; Kenneth Ludmerer, *Genetics and American Society: A Historical Appraisal* (Baltimore, Md.: Johns Hopkins University Press, 1972).

60. Richard Hofstadter, *Social Darwinism in American Thought*, rev. ed. (Boston, Mass.: Beacon Press, 1955 [1944]), ch. 9; Paul Boller, *American Thought in Transition: The Impact of Evolutionary Naturalism, 1865–1900* (Chicago: Rand McNally, 1969), ch. 9.

61. See Roger Smith, "The Boundary between Insanity and Criminal Responsibility in Nineteenth-Century England," in Scull, *Madhouses, Mad-Doctors, and Madmen*, 363–84; idem, "Mental Disorder, Criminal Responsibility, and the Social History of Theories of Volition," *Psychological Medicine* 9, no. 1 (1979): 13–19; idem, *Trial by Medicine: Insanity and Responsibility in Victorian Trials* (Edinburgh: Edinburgh University Press, 1981); Rosenberg, *Trial of the Assassin Guiteau*; Gay Weber, "Science and Society in Nineteenth-Century Anthropology," *History of Science* 12, no. 4 (1974): 273–5.

62. Wolfgang, "Cesare Lombroso," 245.

63. Quoted in Peter Scott, "Henry Maudsley, 1835–1918," in Mannheim, *Pioneers in Criminology*, 212.

64. Henry Mudsley, *The Physiology and Pathology of Mind* (London: Macmillan, 1867); idem, *Responsibility in Mental Disease* (London: Macmillan, 1874).

65. Aubrey Lewis, "Henry Maudsley: His Life and Influence," *Journal of Mental Science* 97 (April 1951): 259–77; H. McIlwain, *Maudsley, Mott, and Mann on the Chemical Physiology and Pathology of the Mind* (London: Institute of Psychiatry, Maudsley Hospital, 1955). pp. 3–16.

66. Maudsley, *Pathology of Mind*, 114, 109.

67. McIlwain, *Maudsley, Mott, and Mann*, 3.

68. Eugene S. Talbot, *Degeneracy: Its Causes, Signs, and Results* (London: Walter Scott Publishing, 1909); Maurice Craig, *Psychological Medicine*, 2nd ed. (Philadelphia, Penn.: B. Blakiston's Son, 1912), pp. 26–7; Charles Folsom, "Mental Diseases," in *A System of Practical Medicine*, ed. William Pepper (Philadelphia, Penn.: Lea Brothers, 1886), vol. 5, pp. 108–15.

69. Hughlings Jackson, "Evolution and Dissolution of the Nervous System," *Popular Science Monthly* (25 June 1884): 171–80; Ackerknecht, *Short History of Psychiatry*, 57.

70. Adolf Meyer, "A Review of the Signs of Degeneracy and Methods of Registration," *AJI* 52 (Jan. 1896): 347. On Meyer see David Rothman, *Conscience and Convenience: The Asylum and its Alternatives in Progressive America* (Boston, Mass.: Little, Brown, 1980), pp. 302–33; Norman Dain, *Clifford W. Beers: Advocate for the Insane* (Pittsburgh, Penn.: University of Pittsburgh Press, 1980), passim; Barbara Sicherman, "The New Psychiatry: Medical and Behavior Science, 1895–1921," in *American Psychoanalysis: Origins and Development*, eds. J. M. Quen and E. T. Carlson (New York: Brunner-Mazel, 1978), pp. 20–37.

71. Comte, *Catechism of Positive Religion*, 222.

72. E. H. Ackerknecht, *Rudolf Virchow* (Madison, Wis.: University of Wisconsin Press, 1953), 204.

73. Darwin, *Expression of Emotions*, 246. See also S. L. Gilman, "Darwin Sees the Insane," *Journal of the History of Behavioral Science* 15, no. 3 (1969): 253–62.

74. Maudsley, *Pathology of Mind,* 109.
75. Hale, *Freud and the Americans,* 75, discusses declining cure rates.
76. See, for example, George M. Beard's view in Rosenberg, "George M. Beard," 253–7, and Bucknill and Tuke, *Manual of Psychological Medicine,* 63.
77. Daniel Hack Tucke, *Insanity in Ancient and Modern Life, with Chapters on its Prevention* (London: Macmillan, 1878), pp. 90–5.
78. Rosenberg, "The Bitter Fruit," 229–35.
79. Ibid., 189–90.
80. The connection between poverty and degeneration theory in French psychiatry during the 1850s is well documented in Marc D. Alexander, "The Administration of Madness and Attitudes towards the Insane in Nineteenth-Century Paris" (Ph.D. dissertation, Johns Hopkins University, 1976), ch. 1.
81. C. Lis and H. Soly, *Poverty and Capitalism in Pre-Industrial Europe* (Hassocks, Sussex: Harvester Press, 1979), pp. 159–89.
82. Louis Chevalier, *Labouring Classes and Dangerous Classes in Paris during the First Half of the Nineteenth Century,* trans. Frank Jellinek (New York: Howard Fertig, 1973 [1958]), pp. 77, 153–4, 359–60, 388–9, 409, 413; Michelle Perrot, "Delinquency and the Penitentiary System in Nineteenth-Century France," in *Deviants and the Abandoned in French Society: Selections from the Annales Economies, Sociétiés, Civilisations,* eds. and trans. E. Forster and P. M. Ranum (Baltimore, Md.: Johns Hopkins University Press, 1978), pp. 225–6, 229–31; Robert Tombs, "Crime and the Security of the State: The 'Dangerous Classes' and Insurrection in Nineteenth-Century Paris," in *Crime and the Law: The Social History of Crime in Western Europe since 1500,* eds. V. A. C. Gatrell et al. (London: Europa Publications, 1980), pp. 215–37.
83. M. J. Cullen, *The Statistical Movement in Early Victorian Britain: The Foundation of Empirical Social Research* (Hassocks, Sussex: Harvester Press, 1979), pp. 71–3, 135–41; David Philips, *Crime and Authority in Victorian England: The Black Country 1835–1860* (London: Croom Helm, 1977), pp. 13–15.
84. E. P. Thompson, "Mayhew and the *Morning Chronicle,*" in *The Unknown Mayhew: Selections from the Morning Chronicle, 1849–1850,* eds. E. P. Thompson and Eileen Yeo (London: Merlin Press, 1971), p. 11.
85. Michael Rose, *The Relief of Poverty, 1834–1914* (London: Macmillan, 1972), p. 15.
86. Thompson, "Mayhew and the *Morning Chronicle,*" 24; H. J. Dyos, "The Slums of Victorian London," *Victorian Studies* 1, no. 11 (1967): 13, 18; Jennifer Davis, "The London Garotting Panic of 1862: A Moral Panic and the Creation of a Criminal Class in Mid-Victorian England," in Gatrell, *Crime and the Law,* 190–213.
87. Gareth Stedman-Jones, *Outcast London: A Study in the Relationship between Classes in Victorian Society* (Oxford: Clarendon Press, 1971), pp. 151, 261, 285–9, 306–7; Pauline Mazumdar, "The Eugenists and the Residuum: The Problem of the Urban Poor," *BHM* 54, no. 2 (1980): 204–15; cf. Victor Bailey, "The Metropolitan Police, The Home Office, and the Threat of Outcast London," in his edited collection, *Policing and Punishment in Nineteenth-Century Britain* (London: Croom Helm, 1981), pp. 94–125.
88. See Michael B. Katz, "Social Class in North American Urban History," *Journal of Interdisciplinary History* 11, no. 4 (1981): 579–605.
89. Robert Bremner, *From the Depths: The Discovery of Poverty in the United States* (New York: New York University Press, 1956), pp. 3–7; Paul Boyer, *Urban Masses and Moral Order in America, 1820–1920* (Cambridge, Mass.: Harvard University Press, 1978), pp. 56, 69.
90. Carl Berger, "The True North Strong and Free," in *Nationalism in Canada,* ed. Peter Russell (Toronto: McGraw-Hill, 1966), pp. 9–12; Judith Fingard, "The Winter's Tale: The Seasonal Contours of Pre-Industrial Poverty in British North America, 1815–1860," Canadian Historical Association, *Historical Papers* (1974): 65–94.
91. Rainer Baehre, "Pauper Emigration to Upper Canada in the 1830s," *Histoire*

Sociale–Social History 15, no. 28 (1981): 339–67; Pat Malcolmson, "The Poor in Kingston, 1815–1850," in *To Preserve and Defend: Essays on Kingston in the Nineteenth Century*, ed. Gerald Tulchinsky (Montreal: McGill University Press, 1976), pp. 281–97.

92. Rainer Baehre, "Paupers and Poor Relief in Upper Canada," Canadian Historical Association, *Historical Papers* (1981): 65–6.

93. Stephen Speisman, "Munificent Parsons and Municipal Parsimony: Voluntary versus Public Relief in Nineteenth-Century Toronto," *Ontario History* 65, no. 1 (1973): 33–49; James Walen, "Social Welfare in New Brunswick, 1784–1900," *Acadiensis* 2, no. 1 (1972): 54–64; Margaret Angus, "Health, Emigration, and Welfare in Kingston, 1820–1840," in *Oliver Mowat's Ontario* (Toronto: Macmillan, 1972), pp. 120–35; Denis Quest, *The Emergence of Social Security in Canada* (Vancouver, B.C.: University of British Columbia Press, 1980), pp. 1–38.

94. Erik Monkkonen, *The Dangerous Class: Crime and Poverty in Columbus, Ohio, 1860–1885* (Cambridge, Mass.: Harvard University Press, 1975).

95. Boyer, *Urban Masses and Moral Order*, 93; Fink, *Causes of Crime. Crime*, passim.

96. Wolfgang, "Cesare Lombroso," 238; R. M. Bucke, *Cosmic Consciousness* (Secaucus, N.J.: Citadel Press, 1977 [1901]), pp. 3–4; Thorstein Sellin, "Enrico Ferri, 1856–1929," in Mannheim, *Pioneers in Criminology*, 373. That degeneration theorists were often social liberals is also noted by Hale, *Freud and the Americans*, 77; Gould, *Ontogeny and Phylogeny*, 121.

97. Gould, *Mismeasure of Man*, 140.

98. On the relation between medical theory and class structure see Donald A. Mackenzie, *Statistics in Britain, 1865–1930: The Social Construction of Scientific Knowledge* (Edinburgh: University of Edinburgh Press, 1981); Roger Cooter, "The Power of the Body: The Early Nineteenth Century," in *Natural Order: Historical Studies of Scientific Culture*, eds. Barry Barnes and Steven Shapin (Beverley Hills, Calif.: Sage Publications, 1979). pp. 73–92; Robert Young, "The Historiographic and Ideological Context of the Nineteenth-Century Debate on Man's Place in Nature," in *Changing Perspectives in the History of Science*, eds. M. Teich and Robert Young (Dordrecht, Netherlands: D. Reidel, 1973), pp. 344–438; idem, "Malthus and the Evolutionists: The Common Context of Biological and Social Theory," *Past and Present* 43 (May 1969): 109–45; Michael S. Helfand, "T. H. Huxley's 'Evolution and Ethics,': The Politics of Evolution and the Evolution of Politics," *Victorian Studies* 20, no. 2 (1977): 519–77; A. R. Buss, "Galton and the Birth of Differential Psychology and Eugenics: Social, Political, and Economic Forces," *Journal of the History of Behavioral Science* 12, no. 1 (1976): 47–58; Garland Allen, "Genetics, Eugenics, and Class Struggle," *Genetics* 79 (1975), Supplement: 29–45; Karl Figlio, "Chlorosis and Chronic Disease in Nineteenth-Century Britain: The Social Constitution of Somatic Illness in a Capitalist Society," *Social History* 3, no. 2 (1978): 167–97.

99. Harvey Simmons, *From Asylum to Welfare: The Evolution of Mental Retardation Policy in Ontario, 1831–1980* (Downsview, Ontario: National Institute on Mental Retardation, 1982), ch. 3 and ch. 4.

100. See Dain, *Clifford W. Beers*, and Haller, *Eugenics*.

101. The printing history is described in M. A. Jameson, ed., *Richard Maurice Bucke: A Catalogue Based upon the Collections of the University of Western Ontario Libraries* (London, Ontario: University of Western Ontario, 1978), pp. 40–1.

102. RMBC, William Osler to Bucke, 24 Sept. 1901; H. B. Forman to Bucke, 22 Sept. 1894; John Harkness to Bucke, 29 May 1892; William James, *The Varieties of Religious Experience: A Study in Human Nature* (New York: Collier Macmillan, 1961), pp. 313–14.

103. RMBC, Bucke to Horace Traubel, 16 Nov. 1891, 21 Feb. 1892, 7 March 1892, 20 March 1892; LC, Feinberg Whitman Collection: Bucke to J. H. Johnston, 6 June 1892; Edward Carpenter to Bucke, 12 April 1893. Carpenter and Bucke shared similar views on a number of topics including socialism, mysticism, and the need for open discussion of sexuality. See Chushichi Tsuzuki, *Edward Car-*

penter, 1844–1929: Prophet of Human Fellowship (New York: Cambridge University Press, 1980), and Sheila Rowbotham and Jeffrey Weeks, *Socialism and the New Life: The Personal and Sexual Politics of Edward Carpenter and Havelock Ellis* (London: Pluto Press, 1970).

104. R. M. Bucke, "Walt Whitman and the Cosmic Sense," in *In Re Walt Whitman*, eds. H. Traubel et al. (Philadelphia, Penn.: David McKay, 1893), pp. 329–47; idem, "Cosmic Consciousness," *Proceedings of the American Medico–Psychological Association* 1 (1894): 316–27; idem, "Mental Evolution in Man," 643–5.

105. RMBC, Bucke to H. B. Forman, 5 Aug. 1898; LC, Feinberg Whitman Collection: Bucke to W. T. Innes, 28 July 1901; Harvard University, Houghton Library Manuscript Collection 6 MS AM 1545: Bucke to Edith Love, 16 Aug. 1901.

106. Bucke, *Cosmic Consciousness*, 21–6, 34, 17, 1–2.

107. Ibid., 8.

108. Ibid., 2.

109. Ibid., 14.

110. Ibid., 56, 317–18.

111. Bucke, "Walt Whitman and the Cosmic Sense," 329.

112. Gay Wilson Allen, *The Solitary Singer, A Critical Biography of Walt Whitman* (New York: Macmillan, 1955), p. 510; Justin Kaplan, *Walt Whitman, A Life* (New York: Simon and Schuster, 1980), p. 35. Cf. Artem Lozynsky, *Richard Maurice Bucke, Medical Mystic: Letters of Dr. Bucke to Walt Whitman and His Friends* (Detroit, Mich.: Wayne State University Press, 1977), pp. 61, 64, 190.

113. Horace Traubel, *With Walt Whitman in Camden* (New York: Rowman and Littlefield, 1961 [1907]), vol. 2, p. 408.

114. Edward Carpenter, *Days with Walt Whitman* (London: George Allen, 1896), p. 37. Carpenter also accepted Bucke's interpretation (see page 55).

115. Though Bucke's letters were an essential phase of his daily routine, Whitman considered them full of "inconsequentials." Horace Traubel, *With Walt Whitman*, ed. Sculley Bradley (n.p.: Southern Illinois Press, 1959), vol. 4, p. 418.

116. Ibid., 6. I have discussed this topic at greater length in "The Myth of a Canadian Boswell: Dr. Richard M. Bucke and Walt Whitman Revisited," *Canadian Bulletin of Medical History* 1, no. 2 (1984): 55–70.

117. J. H. Cassedy, "Hygeia: A Mid-Victorian Dream of a City of Health," *JHMAS* 17, no. 2 (1962): 217–28; Havelock Ellis, *The Nineteenth Century, A Dialogue in Utopia* (London: Grant Richards, 1900). See also George Rosen, "Medicine in Utopia, from the Eighteenth Century to the Present," *Ciba Symposium* 9 (Dec. 1945): 188–200; René Dubois, "Medical Utopias," *Daedalus* 88, no. 3 (1959): 410–24.

118. Austin Flint, "On the Discovery of the Source of the Rochester Knockings, and on Sounds Produced by the Movement of Joints and Tendons," *Quarterly Journal of Medical Science* 3 (1869): 417–46; (editorial), "Spirit Rappers: Physiological Explanation," *AJI* 11 (1855): 294–5.

119. E. C. Rogers, *Philosophy of Mysterious Agents, Human and Mundane: Or, the Dynamic Laws and Relations of Man* (Boston, Mass.: John P. Jewett, 1853); J. Stanley Grimes, *The Mysteries of Human Nature Explained by a New System of Nervous Physiology* (Buffalo, N.Y.: R. M. Wanzer, 1857).

120. I have discussed this theme at greater length in "Physicians and Psychics: The Anglo-American Medical Response to Spiritualism, 1870–1890," *JHMAS* 39, no. 3 (1984): 339–55.

121. Frank Podmore, *Modern Spiritualism: A History and a Criticism* (London: Methuen, 1920), vol. 1, pp. 146–7; Burton G. Brown, "Spiritualism in Nineteenth-Century America," (Ph.D. dissertation, Boston University, 1972), pp. 273–6; Malcolm Kottler, "Alfred Russel Wallace, The Origin of Man, and Spiritualism," *Isis* 65, no. 2 (1974): 145–92; Jon Palfreman, "William Crookes: Spiritualism and Science," *Ethics in Science and Medicine* 3 (1976): 211–27; David Wil-

son, "The Thought of Late-Victorian Physicists: Oliver Lodge's Ethereal Body," *Victorian Studies* 15, no. 1 (1971): 29–48.

122. Brown, "Spiritualism in Nineteenth-Century America," 280; Alan Gauld, *The Founders of Psychical Research* (New York: Schocken Books, 1968), pp. 85–6.

123. A useful summary of the major features of Victorian psychiatric theory is W. F. Bynum, "Themes in British Psychiatry, J. C. Pritchard (1786–1848) to Henry Maudsley (1835–1918)" in *Nature Animated*, ed. Michael Ruse (Dordrecht, Netherlands: D. Reidel, 1983), vol. 2, pp. 225–42.

124. E. L. Margetts, "The Concept of the Unconscious in the History of Medical Psychology," *Psychiatric Quarterly* 27, no. 1 (1953): 133–4; Henri Ellenberger, "The Unconscious before Freud," *Bulletin of the Menninger Clinic* 21, no. 1 (1957): 6–7; L. L. Whyte, *The Unconscious Before Freud* (New York: St. Martin's Press, 1978), pp. 154–5, 163–5.

125. Carpenter, *Principles of Mental Physiology*, 106. Emphasis in the original.

126. Ibid., 674–5. The importance of will as a medical concept is discussed in A. C. Fellman and M. Fellman, *Making Sense of Self: Medical Advice Literature in Late Nineteenth-Century America* (Philadelphia, Penn.: University of Pennsylvania Press, 1981), especially ch. 7.

127. Logie Barrow, "Socialism in Eternity: The Ideology of Plebian Spiritualists, 1853–1913," *History Workshop* 9 (Spring 1980): 37–69; idem, "Anti-establishment Healing: Spiritualism in Britain," in *The Church and Healing* ed. W. J. Sheils (Oxford: Basil Blackwell, 1982), pp. 225–47.

128. Frank M. Turner, "Rainfall, Plagues, and the Prince of Wales: A Chapter in the Conflict of Religion and Science," *Journal of British Studies* 13 (May 1974): 46–65; idem, "The Victorian Conflict between Science and Religion: A Professional Dimension," *Isis* 69 (1978): 356–76.

129. Maudsley, *Pathology of Mind*, 63, 80. Note also his *Natural Causes and Supernatural Seemings*, abridged ed. (London: Watts, 1939 [1886]).

130. George M. Beard, "The Psychology of Spiritualism," *North American Review* 129 (July 1879): 74.

131. W. A. Hammond, *Spiritualism and Allied Causes and Conditions of Nervous Derangement* (New York: G. P. Putnam, 1876), p. 365.

132. Beard, "Psychology of Spiritualism," 70; W. B. Carpenter, *Mesmerism, Spiritualism, Historically and Scientifically Considered* (New York: D. Appleton, 1877), p. 7.

133. Carpenter, *Mesmerism, Spiritualism, ix.*

134. In a slightly different context this dispute has been viewed in part as a confrontation between "certain career scientists and their amateur counterparts." See Jan Palfreman, "Between Spiritualism and Credulity: A Study of Victorian Scientific Attitudes to Modern Spiritualism," in *On the Margins of Science: The Social Construction of Rejected Knowledge* ed. Roy Wallis (Sociological Review Monograph 27, March 1979), pp. 201–36.

135. Gauld, *Founders of Psychical Research*, 140; Samuel Hynes, *The Edwardian Turn of Mind* (Princeton, N.J.: Princeton University Press, 1968), p. 142.

136. Wilson, "Thought of Late Victorian Physicists," passim; P. M. Heimann, "The *Unseen Universe*: Physics and the Philosophy of Nature in Victorian Britain," *British Journal for the History of Science* 6 (June 1972): 73–9; Brian Wynne, "Physics and Psychics: Science, Symbolic Action, and Social Control in Late Victorian England," in Barnes and Shapin, *Natural Order*, 167–86.

137. Gauld, *Founders of Psychical Research*, 64, 91, 141; Hynes, *Edwardian Turn of Mind*, 139, 145; Turner, *Between Science and Religion*, 2–7, 62.

138. Brown, "Spiritualism in Nineteenth-Century America," 312–16; Gauld, *Founders of Psychical Research*, 140.

139. Palfreman, "Between Spiritualism and Credulity," 226–7; James Cerullo, "The Secularization of the Soul: Psychical Research in Britain, 1882–1920," (Ph.D. dissertation, University of Pennsylvania, 1980), pp. 63, 68, 115, 117.

140. Cerullo, "Secularization of the Soul," 128–30; Gauld, *Founders of Psychical Research*, 276; R. Laurence Moore, *In Search of White Crows: Spiritualism, Parapsychology, and American Culture* (New York: Oxford University Press, 1977), pp. 142, 150–3.

141. Henri Ellenberger, *The Discovery of the Unconscious* (New York: Basic Books, 1970), pp. 85–95; Kenneth Levin, *Freud's Early Psychology of Neuroses* (Pittsburgh, Penn.: University of Pittsburgh Press, 1978), pp. 42–51; Ackerknecht, *Short History of Psychiatry*, 84–9; A. R. G. Owen, *Hysteria, Hypnotism, and Healing: The Work of J.-M. Charcot* (New York: Garrett, 1971), ch. 8.

142. Jan Goldstein, "The Hysteria Diagnosis and the Politics of Anticlericalism in Late Nineteenth-Century France," *Journal of Modern History* 54 (June 1982): 236–9; Levin, *Freud's Early Psychology of Neuroses*, 51–3; Sulloway, *Freud*, 48.

143. R. W. Clark, *Freud: The Man and the Cause* (London: Jonathan Cape, 1980), pp. 72–3, 107–8; R. E. Francher, *Pioneers of Psychology* (New York: W. W. Norton, 1979), pp. 193–7.

144. For example, the *American Journal of Insanity* [49 (April 1893): 634–6] reviewed Pierre Janet's *Etat Mental des Hystériques* (Paris: Rueff, n.d.). In contrast to the strict somaticism of earlier decades, the reviewer felt the case had been made that in hysteria "all these symptoms are due to psychical causes rather than to physical lesions" (635).

145. Ross, *G. Stanley Hall*, 164, 174; Seymour Mauskopf and Michael McVaugh, *The Elusive Science: Origins of Experimental Psychical Research* (Baltimore, Md.: Johns Hopkins University Press, 1980), pp. 44, 47; J. B. Rhine, "History of Experimental Study," in *Handbook of Parapsychology*, ed. B. B. Wolman (New York: Van Nostrand Reinhold, 1977), pp. 25–9.

146. Hale, *Freud and the Americans*, 67, 122–3.

147. See, for example, G. Seppilli, "Report on the Therapeusis of Mental Disease by Means of Hypnotic Suggestion," *AJI* 57 (April 1891): 542–56; C. W. Page, "The Relation of Attention to Hypnotic Phenomena," ibid., 47 (July 1891): 27–42; H. S. Smith, "The Dream State and its Psychic Correlatives," ibid., 48 (April 1892): 445–55; C. P. Bancroft, "Subconscious Homicide and Suicide; their Physiological Psychology," ibid., 55 (October 1898): 263–73.

148. William James, "The Hidden Self," *Scribner's Magazine* 7 (March 1890): 361–73.

149. Russell Vasile, *James Jackson Putnam, from Neurology to Psychoanalysis* (New York: Dabor Science Publications, 1977), x–xii; Nathan Hale, ed., *James Jackson Putnam and Psychoanalysis* (Cambridge, Mass.: Harvard University Press, 1971), pp. 11–12; Nathan Hale, "James Jackson Putnam and Boston Neurology, 1877–1918," in *Psychoanalysis, Psychotherapy, and the New England Medical Scene, 1894–1944*, ed. George Gifford (New York: Science History Publications, 1978), pp. 151–3.

150. Otto M. Marx, "Morton Prince and Psychopathology," in Gifford, *New England Medical Scene*, 155–6; "Introduction," Nathan Hale, ed., *Psychotherapy and Multiple Personality: Selected Essays, by Morton Prince* (Cambridge, Mass.: Harvard University Press, 1975), pp. 1–4.

151. Hale, *Freud and the Americans*, 137. See also Sicherman, "New Psychiatry."

152. Cf. James Horne, "R. M. Bucke: Pioneer Psychiatrist, Practical Mystic," *Ontario History* 59, no. 3 (1967): 197–208; idem, "Cosmic Consciousness – Then and Now, The Evolutionary Mysticism of Richard Maurice Bucke," (Ph.D. dissertation, Columbia University, 1964), pp. 25–6, 114, 195.

153. IC, vol. 227, list headed "Medical Books in the London Asylum Library, May 1st, 1902"; *Catalogue of the Library of the Society for Psychical Research* (Boston, Mass.: G. K. Hall, 1976), p. 194.

154. Gauld, *Founders of Psychical Research*, 308; Cerullo, "Secularization of the Soul," 119–20.

155. Bucke, *Cosmic Consciousness*, 304.

156. Bucke, "Mental Evolution in Man," 645. The editors of the *B.M.J.* were very

skeptical of Bucke's position. See *British Medical Journal* 2 (25 Sept. 1897): 827–8.

157. Bucke, "Mental Evolution in Man," 645.

158. Bucke, *Cosmic Consciousness*, 9, 13, 308, 312.

159. See David Armstrong, *Political Anatomy of the Body, Medical Knowledge in Britain in the Twentieth Century* (New York: Cambridge University Press, 1983), ch. 3.

CHAPTER 5 *Treatment tactics and professional aspirations*

1. Nathan Hale, *Freud and the Americans: The Beginnings of Psychoanalysis in the United States, 1876–1917* (New York: Oxford University Press, 1971), ch. 8; David Rothman, *Conscience and Convenience: The Asylum and its Alternatives in Progressive America* (Boston, Mass.: Little, Brown, 1980), pp. 309–12; Gerald Grob, *Mental Illness and American Society, 1875–1940* (Princeton, N.J.: Princeton University Press, 1983), ch. 5 and ch. 6.

2. A. N. Gilbert, "Masturbation and Insanity: Henry Maudsley and the Ideology of Sexual Repression," *Albion* 12, no. 3 (1980): 270–1; E. H. Hare, "Masturbatory Insanity: the History of an Idea," *Journal of Mental Science* 108 (Jan. 1962): 7.

3. G. P. Parsons, "Equal Treatment for All: American Medical Remedies for Male Sexual Problems, 1850–1900," *JHMAS* 31, no. 1 (1977): 63–9; John Duffy, "Masturbation and Clitoridectomy, A Nineteenth-Century View," *Journal of the American Medical Association* 186 (19 Oct. 1963): 246–8; H. T. Engelhardt, Jr., "The Disease of Masturbation: Values and the Concept of Disease," *BHM* 42, no. 2 (1974): 244–5.

4. Hare, "Masturbatory Insanity," 9, 12–15.

5. A. N. Gilbert, "Doctor, Patient, and Onanist Diseases in the Nineteenth Century," *JHMAS* 30, no. 3 (1975): 222–3, 231; Engelhardt, "Disease of Masturbation," 238; Hare, "Masturbatory Insanity," 18; Parsons, "Equal Treatment for All," 70–1.

6. Gilbert, "Masturbation and Insanity," 277; Peter Cominos, "Late-Victorian Sexual Respectability and the Social System," Part 3, *International Review of Social History* 8 (1963): 216, 223; G. J. Barker-Benfield, *The Horrors of the Half-Known Life* (New York: Harper and Row, 1977), pp. 175–88; Caroll Smith-Rosenberg, "Sex as Symbol in Victorian Purity: An Ethnohistorical Analysis of Jacksonian America," *American Journal of Sociology* 84, Supplement (1978): 222; A. C. Fellman and Michael Fellman, *Making Sense of Self: Medical Advice Literature in Late Nineteenth-Century America* (Philadelphia, Penn.: University of Pennsylvania Press, 1981), pp. 92, 106.

7. D. Yellowlees, quoted in "Notes and News," *Journal of Mental Science* 22 (July 1876): 336–7. On Yellowlees see "Notes and Comments," *AJI* 46 (April 1890): 561–3.

8. MSJ, 6 March 1877.

9. MCB, vol. 9. The random sample referred to was chosen from all male patients admitted to the asylum from 1885 to 1900. The twenty-five-year-old clerk is described on page 292.

10. MSJ, 17 July 1877.

11. MCB, vol. 9: 300, 292, 309; MSJ, 1 May 1877; ARMS (1877): 280.

12. Results tabulated from MCB, vol. 9, and compared with ARMS (1877): 280. Bucke appears to have claimed some improvement in five patients in whom the case notes indicate otherwise.

13. ARMS (1877): 279–80. A former assistant shared this view. See Stephen Lett, "The Relationship of Insanity to Masturbation," *Canada Lancet* 20 (19 Aug. 1877): 360–3.

14. IC: vol. 227: "Medical Books in the London Asylum Library, May 1, 1902."

15. A. T. Scull, *Museums of Madness: The Social Organization of Insanity in Nineteenth-Century England* (London: Allen Lane, 1979), p. 183.

198   *Notes to pp. 127–130*

16. ARMS (1884): 68; IR (1895): *xviii*.
17. ARMS (1881): 353–4.
18. Austin Re De Laire, *St. Thomas Evening Journal*, 11 Jan. 1883.
19. For example, ARMS (1877): 279, (1884): 68.
20. ARMS (1897): 42. See J. C. Bucknill and D. H. Tuke, *A Manual of Psychological Medicine* (Philadelphia, Penn.: Blanchard and Lea, 1858 [reprinted New York: Hafner, 1968]), p. 453.
21. Philippe Pinel, *A Treatise on Insanity*, trans. D. D. Davis (Sheffield: Cadell and Davies, 1806); Samuel Tuke, *Description of the Retreat* (York: W. Alexander, 1813).
22. A useful summary of the tenets of moral treatment if found in Ruth B. Caplan, *Psychiatry and the Community in Nineteenth-Century America* (New York: Basic Books, 1969), pp. 29–35; see also J. S. Bockoven, "Moral Treatment in American Psychiatry," *Journal of Nervous and Mental Diseases* 124 (Aug. 1956): 167–94, and (Sept. 1956): 292–321; Eric Carlson and Norman Dain, "The Psychotherapy that Was Moral Treatment," *American Journal of Psychiatry* 117 (Dec. 1960): 519–24; Alexander Walk, "Some Aspects of the 'Moral Treatment' of the Insane up to 1854," *Journal of Mental Science* 100 (Oct. 1954): 807–37.
23. Kathleen Jones, *A History of the Mental Health Services* (London: Routledge and Kegan Paul, 1972), ch. 4. Lawrence quoted in W. F. Bynum, "Rationales for Therapy in British Psychiatry: 1780–1835," *MH* 18, no. 4 (1974): 328.
24. Bynum, "Rationales for Therapy," 322–4; Scull, *Museums of Madness*, 132–41; John Walton, "The Treatment of Pauper Lunatics in Victorian England: The Case of Lancaster Asylum 1816–1870," in *Madhouses, Mad-Doctors and Madmen: The Social History of Psychiatry in the Victorian Era*, ed. A. T. Scull (Philadelphia, Penn.: University of Pennsylvania Press, 1981), pp. 167–8; Eric Carlson, "Amariah Brigham: II, Psychiatric Thought and Practice," *American Journal of Psychiatry* 113 (April 1957): 911–16.
25. Walton, "Treatment of Pauper Lunatics," 191; G. N. Grob, *Mental Institutions in America: Social Policy to 1875* (New York: The Free Press, 1973), pp. 206–10.
26. A. T. Scull, "Moral Treatment Reconsidered: Some Sociological Comments on an Episode in the History of British Psychiatry," *Psychological Medicine* 9, no. 3 (1979): 425. Similar, though less-detailed, observations are found in Vieda Skultans, *English Madness: Ideas on Insanity 1580–1890* (London: Routledge and Kegan Paul, 1978), p. 9, and Caplan, *Psychiatry and the Community*, 26.
27. ARMS (1884): 72.
28. These drugs appear in MCB and FCB and are enumerated in IC: vol. 234: Bucke to J. W. Langmuir, 4 Oct. 1878. A useful summary of popular medications is found in John S. Haller, *American Medicine in Transition, 1840–1910* (Chicago: University of Chicago Press, 1981), ch. 3. See also T. C. Butler, "The Introduction of Chloral Hydrate into Medical Practice," *BHM* 46, no. 2 (1970): 168–72.
29. ARMS (1884): 68.
30. IR (1887): 19. Bucke's approach often corresponded to the pharmaceutical recommendations of Bucknill and Tuke, *Manual of Psychological Medicine*, 458–77, and to the practices current in Irish asylums as described in Mark Finnane, *Insanity and the Insane in Post-Famine Ireland* (London: Croom Helm, 1981), pp. 205–6.
31. Discussed in Thomas E. Brown, " 'Living with God's Afflicted': A History of the Provincial Lunatic Asylum at Toronto, 1830–1911" (Ph.D. dissertation, Queen's University 1980), p. 294.
32. John Harley Warner, "Physiological Theory and Therapeutic Explanation in the 1860s: The British Debate on the Medical Use of Alcohol," *BHM* 54, no. 2 (1980): 235–57.
33. W. B. Carpenter, *Principles of Mental Physiology* (New York: Appleton, 1874), p. 637; Bucknill and Tuke, *Manual of Psychological Medicine*, 358; Benjamin Ward Richardson, *Vita Medica: Chapters of Medical Life and Work* (London:

Longmans, Green & Co., 1897), pp. 364–80; Benjamin W. Richardson, *Diseases of Modern Life* (New York: Appleton, 1895), pp. 209–72.
34. AS: vol. 1: 120, clipping dated 21 Sept. 1893.
35. ARMS (1878): 313, (1882): 70.
36. ARMS (1888): 31–7.
37. W. F. Bynum, "Chemical Structure and Pharmacological Action; A Chapter in the History of Nineteenth-Century Molecular Pharmacology," *BHM* 44, no. 6 (1970): 523–7; John Parascandola, "Structure–Activity Relationships – the Early Mirage," *Pharmacy in History* 13, no. 1 (1971): 5.
38. IR (1887): 37–8.
39. See, for example, A. M. Shew, "Mechanical Restraint," *AJI* 35 (April 1879): 556–62.
40. ARMS (1887): 274.
41. IR (1887): 26, (1868): (1878): 36; ARMS (1884): 71. O'Reilly gave Bucke credit for initiating the nonrestraint system. See IR (1887): 36–7.
42. ARMS (1879): 330.
43. ARMS (1886): 25, (1882): 71; IR (1881): 34.
44. ARMS (1884): 69–72.
45. ARMS (1887): 276, (1881): 28. On *work therapy* in Irish and American asylums respectively, see Finnane, *Insanity and the Insane*, 196–7; Caplan, *Psychiatry and the Community*, 160–7.
46. ARMS (1884): 72, 73, (1883): 85–6. The London Asylum exceeded the other institutions in Ontario in terms of average days worked. See IR (1887): 22.
47. ARMS (1883): 86; IMB: 15 Jan. 1884.
48. Asa Briggs, *Victorian People* (Harmondsworth: Penguin Books, 1965), ch. 5; Walter Houghton, *The Victorian Frame of Mind, 1830–1870* (New Haven, Conn.: Yale University Press, 1957), pp. 242–62. A similar observation is made of English practice in Skultans, *English Madness*, 17.
49. ARMS (1883): 87.
50. ARMS (1883): 87, (1880): 314, (1890): 70; RMBC, Diary (1 Jun. 1878–19 Nov. 1878): 31 Jan. 1878; MSOB, 20 Nov. 1881.
51. ARMS (1885): 66, (1898): 72; RMBC, Diary (1 Jan. 1878–19 Nov. 1878): 4 July 1878; University of Western Ontario: D. B. Weldon Library, Diary of Charles A. Sippi, 1893–1897: 20 July 1893; AS: vol. 1: 5, "Lunatics at the Show," n.d. On recreation in Irish asylums, see Finnane, *Insanity and the Insane*, 197–8.
52. Finnane, *Insanity and the Insane*, 200–1; Caplan, *Psychiatry and the Community*, 35–6.
53. ARMS (1896): 75.
54. R. M. Bucke, *Cosmic Consciousness, A Study in the Evolution of the Human Mind* (Secaucus, N.J.: Citadel Press, 1977 [1901]), dedication, in which he professes a belief in an afterlife.
55. ARMS (1880): 310; MSJ, 12 Sept. 1880.
56. ARMS (1887): 69, (1877): 275; MSOB, 25 Oct. 1880.
57. LC, Feinberg Whitman Collection, Bucke to Whitman, 24 Sept. 1888; MSJ, 28 Sept. 1877; IC: vol. 227: D. M. McCallum to Robert Christie, 14 Aug. 1902; Christie to McCallum, 15 Aug. 1902.
58. ARMS (1892): 40; Sippi Diary: 7 Sept. 1892; MSJ, 23 April 1879, 10 Sept. 1879; IC: vol. 73: Bucke to Robert Christie, 10 May 1901.
59. D. H. Tuke visited and published his impressions in *The Insane in the United States and Canada* (London: H. K. Lewis, 1885), pp. 217–26. Henry Hurd, who also came in 1884, later published his views in *The Institutional Care of the Insane in the United States and Canada* (Baltimore, Md.: Johns Hopkins University Press, 1916–17).
60. *London (Ontario) Free Press*, 1 Oct. 1878. Bucke condemned this paper in print (AS: vol. 1: 57–8, clipping, no source or date) and rightly informed the Inspector that it printed anything "adverse to the asylum" (IC: vol. 224: Bucke to Robert Christie, 11 Jan. 1899).

61. ARMS (1884): 68.
62. ARMS (1890): 68.
63. E. H. Ackerknecht, *Medicine at the Paris Hospital* (Baltimore, Md.: Johns Hopkins University Press, 1967), ch. 11; Jacob Bigelow, *Discourse on Self-Limited Diseases* (Boston, Mass.: Nathan Hale, 1835); Elisha Bartlett, *An Essay on the Philosophy of Medical Science* (Philadelphia, Penn.: Lea and Blanchard, 1844): Oliver Wendell Holmes, *Currents and Counter-Currents in Medical Science* (Boston, Mass.: Ticknor and Fields, 1860).
64. Gert H. Brieger, "Therapeutic Conflicts and the American Medical Profession in the 1860s," *BHM* 41, no. 3 (1967): 215–22; Leon Bryan, "Blood-letting in American Medicine, 1830–1892," *BHM* 38, no. 6 (1964): 516–29; Martin Kaufman, *Homeopathy in America: The Rise and Fall of a Medical Heresy* (Baltimore, Md.: Johns Hopkins University Press, 1971); John Harley Warner, " 'The Nature-Trusting Heresy': American Physicians and the Concepts of the Healing Power of Nature in the 1850s and 1860s," *Perspectives in American History* (Cambridge, Mass.: Harvard University Press, 1978), vol. 11, pp. 291–324.
65. William Paton, "The Evolution of Therapeutics: Osler's Therapeutic Nihilism and the Changing Pharmacopoeia," *Journal of the Royal College of Physicians of London* 13, no. 2 (1979): 74–83; Holmes, *Currents and Counter-Currents*.
66. Frederick Tilney and Smith Ely Jelliffe, *Semi-Centennial Anniversary Volume of the American Neurological Association, 1875–1924* (Albany N.Y.: American Neurological Association, 1924), pp. 1, 29, 35, 38. See R. N. DeJong, *A History of American Neurology* (New York: Raven Press, 1982), pp. 14–62, for biographical sketches of leading American neurologists of the late nineteenth century.
67. Barbara Sicherman, *The Quest for Mental Health in America, 1880–1917* (New York: Arno Press, 1980), pp. 38, 159, 174, 176, 182.
68. Cited in John A. Pitts, "The Association of Medical Superintendents of American Institutions for the Insane, 1844–1892: A Case Study of Specialism in American Medicine" (Ph.D. dissertation, University of Pennsylvania, 1979), p. 159.
69. Ibid., 188, 192–3, 203, 210, 214, 218.
70. S. Weir Mitchell, "Address before the Fiftieth Annual Meeting of the American Medico–Psychological Association, Held in Philadelphia, May 16th, 1894," *Journal of Nervous and Mental Disease* 21, no. 7 (July 1894): 414, 415, 418, 420.
71. Ibid., 418, 424, 429.
72. Ibid., 422.
73. Pitts, "Association of Medical Superintendents," 221–2; Sicherman, *Quest for Mental Health*, 252.
74. ARMS (1896): 79; IR (1895): *xxii*.
75. R. M. Bucke, *Man's Moral Nature* (New York: J. P. Putnam's Sons, 1879), pp. 51, 96; A. T. Hobbs, "Gynecology among the Insane," *Canadian Practitioner* 21, no. 5 (1896): 321; idem, "Resumé of the Gynecological Work Done at the London Asylum," *American Journal of Obstetrics* 35, no. 3 (1897): 1.
76. E. G. T. Liddell, *The Discovery of Reflexes* (Oxford: Clarendon Press, 1960), ch. 1 and ch. 2; Franklin Fearing, *Reflex Action: A Study in the History of Physiological Psychology* (New York: Hafner, 1964), ch. 5 and ch. 9; J. P. Swazey, *Reflexes and Motor Integration: Sherrington's Concept of Integrative Action* (Cambridge, Mass.: Harvard University Press, 1969), ch. 2; M. P. Amacher, "Thomas Laycock, I. M. Sechenov, and the Reflex Arc Concept," *BHM* 38, no. 2 (1964): 168–83.
77. W. B. Carpenter, *Principles of Human Physiology* (Philadelphia, Penn.: Blanchard and Lea, 1855), pp. 543, 629; R. B. Todd and William Bowman, *The Physiological Anatomy and Physiology of Man* (London: John W. Parker and Son, 1856), vol. 1, pp. 387–8, 392.
78. L. S. Jacyna, "Somatic Theories of Mind and the Interests of Medicine in Britain, 1850–1879," *MH* 26, no. 3 (1982): 240.
79. Bucknill and Tuke, *Manual of Psychological Medicine*, 382.

80. Henry Maudsley, *The Pathology of Mind* (London: Macmillan, 1879), p. 206.

81. Indicative of the growing discontent with the vague notion of "reflex action" was the skepticism of the American neurologist, Edward Spitzka in his *Insanity: its Classification, Diagnosis, and Treatment* (New York: E. B. Treat, 1889), pp. 112–13. On the general retreat from what Adolf Meyer referred to as the "neurologizing fallacy" in psychiatry, see Barbara Sicherman, "The New Psychiatry: Medical and Behavioral Science, 1895–1921" in *American Psychoanalysis: Origins and Development*, eds. J. M. Quen and E. T. Carlson (New York: Brunner-Mazel, 1978), pp. 20–37, and Hale, *Freud and the Americans*, ch. 23.

82. Carpenter, *Principles of Mental Physiology*, 660; Hale, *Freud and the Americans*, ch. 4.

83. Thomas Allbutt and W. S. Playfair, eds., *A System of Gynaecology* (London: Macmillan, 1896), pp. 225–30; Matthew D. Mann, ed., *A System of Gynecology by American Authors* (Philadelphia, Penn.: Lea Brothers, 1888), pp. 59, 82–4. Insanity related to pregnancy, the birth process, or lactation was also a widely accepted diagnosis. See, for example, Barton Hirst, ed., *A System of Obstetrics by American Authors* (Philadelphia, Penn.: Lea Brothers, 1889), pp. 545–632. Popular monographs included Isaac Baker-Brown, *On the Curability of Certain Forms of Insanity, Epilepsy, Catalepsy, and Hysteria in Females* (London: Robert Hardwicke, 1866); Horatio Storer, *The Cause, Course, and Treatment of Reflex Insanity in Women* (Boston: Lee and Shephard, 1871).

84. Bucknill and Tuke, *Manual of Psychological Medicine*, 258; Maudsley, *Pathology of Mind*, 208, 211, 214, 218–19.

85. G. J. Barker-Benfield, *The Horrors of the Half-Known Life* (New York: Harper and Row, 1977), p. 83. Norman Dain, *Concepts of Insanity in the United States, 1789–1865* (New Brunswick, N.J.: Rutgers University Press, 1964), p. fn. 28; S. Weir Mitchell, *Lectures of Diseases of the Nervous System, Especially in Women* (Philadelphia, Penn.: Henry C. Lea's Son, 1881), pp. 224–6; Spitzka, *Insanity*, 376–7.

86. R. M. Bucke, "Gynecological Notes," *American Medico–Psychological Association Proceedings* 3 (1896): 159–60, 141.

87. R. M. Bucke quoted in "Proceedings of the Association," *AJI* 49 (Oct. 1892): 248. On conservative treatment see, for example, FCB, 3: 128, 205; 4: 154.

88. ARMS (1895): 44–5; Bucke, "Gynecological Notes," 158–9.

89. ARMS (1896): 82–5, (1897): 44–51, (1898): 76–81, (1899): 73–5, (1900): 36–40.

90. ARMS (1899): 70.

91. Hobbs, "Gynecological Work Done at the London Asylum," 4.

92. ARMS (1897): 42.

93. R. M. Bucke, "Surgery among the Insane in Canada," *American Medico–Psychological Association Proceedings* 5 (1898): 84, 86, 87.

94. IC: vol. 220: A. T. Hobbs to R. M. Bucke, 26 March 1895.

95. A. T. Hobbs, "Surgical Gynaecology in Insanity," *British Medical Journal* 2 (25 Sept. 1897): 769; idem, "Surgery among the Insane: Its Difficulties, its Advantages, its Results," *The Canadian Journal of Medicine and Surgery* 8, no. 1 (July 1900): 2; Bucke, "Surgery among the Insane," 78.

96. Richard Wertz and Dorothy Wertz, *Lying-In: A History of Childbirth in America* (New York: Schocken Books, 1979), pp. 108–11; Jean Donnison, *Midwives and Medical Men* (New York: Shocken Books, 1977), pp. 187–90.

97. J. Ian Casselman, " 'The Secret Plague': Venereal Disease in Early Twentieth-Century Canada" (M.A. thesis, Queen's University, 1981), ch. 4.

98. C. Frederic Fluhmann, "The Rise and Fall of Suspension Operations for Uterine Retrodisplacements," *Bulletin of the Johns Hopkins Hospital* 96 (1956): 60, 63, 64; Harold Spreet, "John Clarence Webster, John Montgomery Baldy, and their Operations for Uterine Retroversion," *Surgery, Gynecology, and Obstetrics* 102, no. 3 (March 1956): 377.

99. All data has been tabulated from FMC, vols. 2–6.

100. ARMS (1900): 34; R. M. Bucke, "Two Hundred Operative Cases – Insane

Women," *Proceedings of the American Medico–Psychological Association* 7 (1900): 101.

101. H. K. Beecher, "Surgery as Placebo," *Journal of the American Medical Association* 176 (1 July 1961): 1102–7; Lester Lubrorsky, et al., "Factors Influencing the Outcome of Psychotherapy: A Review of Quantitative Research," *Psychological Bulletin* 75, no. 3 (1971): 145–85; W. A. Anthony, et al., "Efficacy of Psychiatric Rehabilitation," *Psychological Bulletin* 78, no. 6 (1980): 447–56.

102. James Russell, "The After-Effects of Surgical Procedures on Generative Organs of Females for the Relief of Insanity," *British Medical Journal* 2 (25 Sept. 1897): 771, 774; ARMS (1889): 72, 76; A. T. Hobbs, "Surgical Gynecology among the Insane: Right or Wrong?" *Canadian Practitioner* 24, no. 7 (1899): 380–1; Daniel Clark, "Reflexes in Psychiatry," *British Medical Journal* 2 (25 Sept. 1897): 780; ARMS (1898): 75, (1896): 79; Bucke, "Two Hundred Operative Cases," 102.

103. Discussion following Bucke, "Gynecological Notes," 147–60; "Annual Meeting: The Sections, Psychology," *British Medical Journal* 2 (18 Sept. 1897): 724; Hobbs, "Surgical Gynecology among the Insane," 379; ARMS (1900).

104. Bucke, "Surgery among the Insane," 75; Sippi Diary: 8 Oct. 1897; IC: vol. 223: Robert Christie to C. K. Clarke, 2 Feb. 1899.

105. G. H. Rohe, "Proceedings of the Association," *AJI* 49 (Oct. 1892): 235–8; idem, "The Etiological Relation of Pelvic Disease in Women to Insanity," *British Medical Journal* 2 (25 Sept. 1897): 766–9. See also Robert A. Kitto, "Ovariotomy as a Prophylaxis and Cure for Insanity," *Journal of the American Medical Association* 16 (11 April 1891): 516–17; and I. S. Stone, "Psychical Results of Gynecological Operations," ibid., 15 (30 Aug. 1890): 305–7.

106. E. A. Hall, "Gynecological Treatment in the Insane," *Canadian Practitioner* 33, no. 3 (1908): 147–51; idem, "Melancholia versus Ovarian Cystoma," *Canadian Lancet* 38, no. 10 (1905): 904–5; idem, "Experiences in the Treatment of Pelvic Diseases in the Female Insane," *Canada Lancet* 37, no. 3 (1903): 301–12. During the 1890s Hall had been one of Bucke's few Canadian supporters. See his "The Surgical Treatment of the Insane in Private Practice," *Dominion Medical Monthly* 12, no. 1 (1899): 1–18; idem, "Pelvic Disease and Insanity," *Canadian Medical Review* 8, no. 4 (1898): 105–14. Another supporter was A. L. Smith, "Insanity in Women from the Gynecological and Obstetric Point of View," *Canada Lancet* 34, no. 12 (1901): 655–63.

107. I. S. Stone, "Can the Gynecologist Aid the Alienist in Institutions for the Insane?" *Journal of the American Medical Association* 16 (20 June 1891): 870–3; Russell, "Ater-Effects of Surgical Procedures," 772–4.

108. Discussion following Bucke, "Gynecological Notes," 147–60; "Annual Meeting, the Sections, Psychology," (1897), 724; J. B. Fleming, "Clitoridectomy – The Disastrous Downfall of Isaac Baker-Brown, F.R.C.S. (1867)," *Journal of Obstetrics and Gynecology of the British Empire* 67, no. 6 (1960): 1017–34.

109. IC: vol. 223: Bucke to Robert Christie, 15 Feb. 1897, enclosure, typed copy of a resolution dated 12 Feb. 1897 over the signature of W. English, secretary of the London Medical Association; *London News* 16 Feb. 1897.

110. RMBC, unsigned typed draft of a letter dated 16 Nov. 1897; Bucke, "Surgery among the Insane," 75; cf. slightly different numerical results in IC: vol. 223: typescript headed "opinion of Doctors in the London Asylum District,"

111. IC: vol. 223: C. K. Clarke to Robert Christie, 1 Feb. 1899, with typed précis of the circular to the local branches of the National Council of Women. The National Council of Women had a dynamic interest in health issues, including insanity. See Rosa Shaw, *Proud Heritage: A History of the National Council of Women in Canada* (Toronto: Ryerson, 1957), pp. 37–75; V. Strong-Boag, *The Parliament of Women: The National Council of Women in Canada, 1893–1929* (Ottawa: National Museums of Canada, 1976), p. 204.

112. See, for example, RMBC, Diary (12 March 1863–7 Dec. 1864): 12 March 1863; and Diary (8 Dec. 1864–19 Oct. 1868): 10 March 1865.

113. Cf. Ann Douglas Wood, " 'The Fashionable Disease': Women's Complaints and Their Treatment in Nineteenth-Century America," *Journal of Interdisciplinary History* 4, no. 1 (1973): 25–52; Barker-Benfield, *Horrors of the Half-Known Life,* passim.

114. Hobbs, "Surgical Gynecology among the Insane," 382.

115. ARMS (1897): 42; Hobbs, "Gynecological Work Done at the London Asylum," 1; idem, "Surgical Gynecology Among the Insane," 381, 382, 383; idem, "Gynecology Among the Insane," 323. Similar views on modernization were expressed in Hall, "Pelvic Disease and Insanity," 113, and idem, "Surgical Treatment of the Insane," 18.

116. Cited in W. B. Beacham, "History of the Section on Obstetrics and Gynecology of the American Medical Association," *Journal of the American Medical Association* 169, no. 13 (1959): 143. On antisepsis in Anglo-American medicine see: A. J. Youngson, *The Scientific Revolution in Victorian Medicine* (London: Croom Helm, 1979), ch. 5; Gert Brieger, "American Surgery and the Germ Theory of Disease," *BHM* 40, no. 2 (1966): 135–45; J. T. H. Connor, "Joseph Lister's System of Wound Management and the Canadian Medical Practitioner, 1867–1900" (M.A. thesis, University of Western Ontario, 1980).

117. H. S. Taylor and E. S. Taylor, "The History of the American Gynecological Society and the Scientific Contributions of its Fellows," *American Journal of Obstetrics and Gynecology* 126, no. 7 (1976): 908; A. F. Lash, "History of Gynecology from Prehistoric to Modern Times," *Journal of the International College of Surgery* 32, no. 6 (1959): 572; W. R. Winterton, "The Story of the London Gynaecological Hospitals," *Proceedings of the Royal Society of Medicine* 54 (March 1961): 194; H. E. MacDermott, *A History of the Montreal General Hospital* (Montreal: Montreal General Hospital, 1950), p. 94; Margaret Angus, *Kingston General Hospital: A Social and Institutional History* (Montreal: McGill-Queen's University Press for Kingston General Hospital, 1973), p. 72; W. G. Crosbie, *The Toronto General Hospital, 1819–1965: A Chronicle* (Toronto: Macmillan, 1975), p. 134.

118. G. H. Lyman, *The History and Statistics of Ovariotomy* (Boston, Mass.: John Wilson, 1856); John Woodward, *To Do the Sick No Harm: A Study of the British Voluntary Hospital System to 1875* (London: Routledge and Kegan Paul, 1974), pp. 81–2; J. A. Shephard, *Spencer Wells* (Edinburgh: E. and S. Livingston, 1965), ch. 5 and ch. 6; idem, *Lawson Tait, the Rebellious Surgeon* (Lawrence, Kans.: Coronado Press, 1980), ch. 4; J. Willocks, "Pioneers of Ovarian Surgery," *Surgo* 7, no. 2 (1970): 5–8; D. Longo, "The Rise and Fall of Battey's Operation: A Fashion in Surgery," *BHM* 53, no. 2 (1979): 244–67.

119. L. A. Enge and R. B. Durfee, "Pelvic Organ Prolapse: Four Thousand Years of Treatment," *Clinical Obstetrics and Gynecology* 9, no. 4 (1966): 1008; J. V. Ricci, *One Hundred Years of Gynecology, 1800–1900* (Philadelphia, Penn.: Blakiston, 1945), p. 335.

120. Fluhmann, "Rise and Fall of Suspension Operations," 63; C. Danielson, "History and Review of the Literature on Prolapse of the Uterus and Vagina," *Acta Obstetrics et Gynecologica Scandinavia* 36, Supplement 1 (1957): 18–25.

121. Ricci, *One Hundred Years of Gynecology,* ch. 8.

122. Bucke, "Surgery among the Insane," 87. Note Hobbs's combination of reflex action and internal secretion in "Surgery among the Insane," 5.

123. Cited in Merriley Barell, "Setting the Standards for a New Science: Edward Schafer and Endocrinology," *MH* 22, no. 2 (1978): fn. 17.

124. Robert Kohler, *From Medical Chemistry to Biochemistry* (New York: Cambridge University Press, 1982), esp. ch. 7; idem, "Medical Reform and Biomedical Science: Biochemistry – A Case Study," in *The Therapeutic Revolution: Essay in the Social History of American Medicine,* eds. M. J. Vogel and C. E. Rosenberg (Philadelphia, Penn.: University of Pennsylvania Press, 1979), pp. 27–66.

125. Merriley Borell, "Organotherapy, British Physiology, and the Discovery of the Internal Secretions," *Journal of the History of Biology* 9, no. 2 (1976): 235–68;

idem, "Brown-Séguard's Organotherapy and its Appearance in America at the End of the Nineteenth Century," *BHM* 50, no. 3 (1976): 309–20; Victor C. Medvei, *A History of Endocrinology* (Lancaster, Penn.: MTP Press, 1982), ch. 16; C. M. Brooks, "The Beginnings of Endocrinology and the Discovery of the Digestive System Hormones," in *Humors, Hormones, and Neurosecretions*, eds. C. M. Brooks et al. (New York: State University of New York Press, 1962), pp. 21–39.

126. T. E. Brown, "Shell Shock in the Canadian Expeditionary Force, 1914–1918: Canadian Psychiatry and the Great War," in *Health, Disease, and Medicine: Essays in Canadian History*, ed. Charles Roland (Toronto: Clark Irwin, 1984); Stephen Jay Gould, *The Mismeasure of Man* (New York: W. W. Norton, 1981), pp. 192–234.

INDEX

alcohol, dispute over medicinal use, 129–
30
alienists: assistant asylum physicians, 33–
4; critisized by neurologists, 139–40;
and degeneration theory, 103–4, 123;
isolation of, 161–2; loss of medical
identity, 35, 41–2; public image, 140–
1; therapeutic frustration, 124, 127,
138; threatened status, 155
American Journal of Insanity, 2, 80, 95, 121,
127, 140
American Medico-Psychological Association, 2, 111, 153, 154; *see also* Association of Medical Superintendents of
American Institutions for the Insane
American Psychoanalytic Association, 122
Association of Medical Superintendents of
American Institutions for the Insane,
139–40; *see also* American Medico-
Psychological Association
associationist psychology, 75, 84–5, 86
asylums Ontario: cost of, 39–40; growth
of, 26; overcrowding, 38–9; patronage in , 41
atavism 98, 100; *see also* degeneration
attendants, asylum, 43–9

Bain, Alexander, 84–5, 87, 88, 89, 90
Baker-Brown, Isaac, 142
Battey, Robert, 156
Beard, George M., 96, 115, 118, 139
Beau, Joseph, 14
Bichat, Xavier, 76, 79, 87, 88
Boston School, 121
British Medical Association, 2, 111, 122,
153, 154
Bucke, Richard Maurice: asylum appoint-
ment, 24; asylum therapeutics, 127–
37; and atheism, 63, 66, 134–5; career,
1–2; childhood and adolescence, 5–6;
Cosmic Consciousness, 109–15, 122–3;
etiology of insanity, 97–9; general
practice, 18–21; gynecological surgery

program, 143–58; illumination, 23;
Man's Moral Nature 79, 85–91; McGill
thesis, 66, 68–70; medical school, 6–
10; medical superintendent position,
32–6; on medicinal use of alcohol,
129–30; on mental evolution, 97, 111;
panic attacks, 21–3; and positivism,
71–7; postgraduate training, 10–16;
and spiritualism, 122–3; study of sympathetic nervous system, 79, 85–8;
treatment of masturbatory insanity,
125–7
Bucknill, John C., 95, 125, 128, 129, 142
Burgess, T. J., 34
Burrows, George Man, 96

Carpenter, Edward, 91, 111, 113, 154
Carpenter, W. B., 91, 114, 115, 129; on
associationism, 86; on correlation of
vital forces, 68–70; on evolution of
nervous system, 89, 90; on mental pathology, 95; on reflex action, 141–2;
on spiritualism, 118; on Will, 117
cerebral localization, 74, 83–4, 86
Chambers, Robert 5, 97
Charcot, J.-M., 101, 120, 122
Clark, Daniel, 129, 152
Clarke, C. K., 154
Comte, Auguste, 71, 72, 73, 74–7, 85, 86,
87, 89, 90, 98, 114; *see also* positivism
Conolly, John, 43, 96, 128
criminology, 101–3
Crookes, William, 115, 118

Darwin, Charles, 4, 77, 91, 97, 98, 103,
115
Davey, J. G., 79, 86, 88
degeneration, doctrine of, 100–9, 161; *see
also* atavism
drugs, therapeutic role of, 129

Ecole de Médicine, Paris, 14
Ellis, Havelock, 102, 114, 125

endocrinology, 157–8
environment, etiological role in Bucke's view of insanity, 90
evolution, doctrine of: applied to neurology, 86, 89–90, 97; as stated by Auguste Comte, 76; *see also* atavism; degeneration

Fergusson, William, 11
forces, doctrine of correlation of, 66–8
Forman, Alfred, 71, 91
Forman, Henry, 13, 14, 24, 71, 72, 77–8, 79, 91, 110, 111
Freud, Sigmund, 99, 111, 118, 119, 120, 122, 124, 162

Gall, Franz Joseph, 74, 76, 83–4, 85, 102
Galton, Francis, 97
Geiger, Lazarus, 98
general practice, 18–21
Grey, John P., 95
Grove, W. R., 68, 69
gynecology: disorders as cause of insanity, 142–3; and doctrine of reflex action, 142; lack of favor among Victorian alienists, 152; London Asylum use of, 143–51; rise of specialty after 1870, 155–7

Haeckel, Ernst, 89, 98, 99
Hall, Ernest, 153
Hall, George Stanley, 99, 119, 121
Hall, Marshall, 141
Hall, Robert Gardiner, 128
Hammond, W. A., 116, 118, 139
heredity, 89–90, 96, 98, 99; *see also* ativism; degeneration
Hillier, Thomas, 12
Hobbs, A. T., 34, 141, 143–6, 152, 154
Holmes, Oliver Wendell, 138
homeopathy, 138
Howard, R. Palmer, 9
Hurd, Henry, 2
Hutchinson, Jonathan, 12
hypnosis, 120

insanity: as degeneration, 100–9; etiological views, 95–6; incurable, 127; pelvic pathology cause of, 142–3; treatment of, 127–37
Inspector of Prisons and Public Charities, 36–40; opposition to gynecological treatment of insane women, 153

Jackson, John Hughlings, 13, 103, 161
James, William, 23, 109, 118, 119, 120, 121

Janet, Pierre, 111, 118, 119, 120, 122, 162
Jarvis, Edward, 143
Jenner, Sir William, 11, 21, 22, 24
Jung, Carl Gustav, 120

King's College Hospital, London, 11

Landor, Henry, 48
Langmuir, J. W., 34, 37, 131
Laycock, Thomas, 116, 141
Lett, Stephen, 33
Lombroso, Cesare, 99, 101–3, 108, 118, 127, 161
London Asylum: admissions, 50–2; architecture, 28; assistant physicians, 33–4; attendants, 43–9; attendant and patient subculture, 49, 58–9; bureaucratic structure, 42; classification of patients, 57–8; discharges, 60–1; gynecological surgery at, 143–51; Inspector of Prisons and Public Charities, 36–40; interior of, 30–1; medical superintendent, 32–6; opposition to gynecological surgery, 152–3; patients, 49–61; poverty of patients, 55–7; structural flaws, 30; support for gynecological surgery, 154; treatment at, 127–37
Lucas, Prosper, 100
Lyell, Charles, 97

Magnan, Valentin, 101, 103
masturbatory insanity, 125–7
Maudsley, Henry, 36, 79, 95, 96, 98, 102, 104, 115, 117, 125, 142
Mayhew, Henry, 106
McGill University, Faculty of Medicine, 6–10
medical profession: in Ontario, 16–18; scientific authority of, 92–3
medical psychology, 117–18, 120–2, 160; *see also* psychiatry, Victorian
mental hygiene movement, 124, 141, 162
Meryon, Edward, 79, 86
Meyer, Adolf, 103, 121
Mill. J. S., 72, 84–5
Mitchell, Silas Weir, 2, 35, 42, 139–40, 143
Montreal General Hospital, 8
moral sense, 76–7, 85–91
moral treatment, 128–9
Moreau de Tours, Jacques, 100, 106
Morel, Benedict, 101, 102, 103, 106
Müller, Johannes, 141
Müller, Max, 97
Myers, Frederick, 119, 122

National Council of Women, 154
neurology, 121, 139–40; *see also Mitchell, Silas Weir; Spitzka, Edward*

O'Reilly, W. T., 35, 37, 131
Osler, Sir William, 2, 109, 138

Pardee, Thomas, 24
Paris: medical education in, 14–16
Paris Clinical School, 15, 138
patients, asylum: characteristics of, 49–61; treatment of, 127–37
philology, 97, 98
physiology: changes in 1870s, 70–1
Pinel, Philippe, 128
positivism, 72–7, 160; *see also* Comte, Auguste
poverty: in the asylum, 55–7; and etiology of insanity, 105–9
Prince, Morton, 120, 121, 122
psychiatry, Victorian: dispute with neurologists, 139–40; factors determining character of, 3; lags behind medicine and surgery, 138, 162; moves beyond the asylum, 159, 162; search for new treatments and theories, 155–8; theoretical upheaval, 121–2; vulnerability of, 117–18; *see also* alienists; *see also* medical psychology
psychical research, 120–2
Putnam, James Jackson, 121, 122

Quain, Richard, 11

Ray, Isaac, 96, 143
recapitulation, doctrine of, 89, 98, 99, 100
recreation, therapeutic role of, 133–4
reflex action, doctrine of, 141–3, 158
religion, therapeutic role of, 134–6
restraint, use in asylums, 128–9, 130–1
Reynolds, John Russell, 12, 72, 79
Richardson, Sir Benjamin Ward, 2, 13, 24, 72, 79, 80, 87, 91, 114, 130
Rohe, George H., 153

Romanes, J. G., 97, 112
Royal London Ophthalmic Hospital, 12
Russell, James, 152

Schafer, Edward, 157
science, Victorian: and religion, 63–4, 92
Sharpey, William, 11
Sims, J. Marion, 156
Sippi, Charles, 33
Society for Psychical Research, 118–22
Spencer, Herbert, 72, 84–5, 98
spiritualism 115–22
Spitzka, Edward, 35, 96, 125, 139, 143
Stone, I. S., 153
surgery, Victorian, 138; *see also* gynecology
sympathetic nervous system, 78–9, 87
sympathy, *see* reflex action

Tait, Lawson, 156
therapeutic pessimism, 127, 138, 160
therapy, asylum: pessimism about, 127; social message of, 137–8; theoretical basis, 138; varieties of, 127–36
Thompson, Sir Henry, 11
Traubel, Horace, 35, 111
Trousseau, Armand, 14–16
Tuke, Daniel Hack, 2, 36, 88, 95, 104, 125, 127, 128, 142
Tuke, Samuel, 128

unconscious, 109, 120–2, 162
Universalism, 64–6, 89, 91, 114
University College Hospital, London, 11
utopianism, medical, 113–14

Virchow, Rudolf, 4, 103
vitalism, 66

Wallace, Alfred Russel, 115, 118
Wells, Spencer, 13, 156
Whitman, Walt, 35, 90, 91, 109, 110, 111, 112, 113, 154
work therapeutic role of, 131–3